M. Steven Piver MD

Deputy Chief (Gynecology), Clinical Professor,
Department of Gynecologic Oncology, Roswell Park
Memorial Institute, Buffalo, New York

Ovarian Malignancies:

The Clinical Care of Adults and Adolescents

With a chapter on the Pathology of Ovarian Tumours by
Robert E. Scully MD
Professor of Pathology, Harvard Medical School,
Massachusetts General Hospital, Boston

Series Editors
ALBERT SINGER AND JOE JORDAN

Churchill Livingstone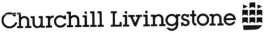

EDINBURGH LONDON MELBOURNE AND NEW YORK 1983

CHURCHILL LIVINGSTONE
Medical Division of Longman Group Limited

Distributed in the United States of America by Churchill
Livingstone Inc., 1560 Broadway, New York, N.Y.
10036, and by associated companies, branches and
representatives throughout the world.

First published 1983

ISBN 0 443 02553 3

British Library Cataloguing in Publication Data
Piver, M. Steven
    Ovarian malignancies. — (Current reviews in obstetrics
    and gynaecology; 4)
    1. Ovaries — Cancer
    I. Title   II. Series
    618.1'105   RC280.08

Library of Congress Cataloging in Publication Data
Piver, M. Steven.
    Ovarian malignancies.
    (Current reviews in obstetrics and gynaecology; 4)
    Includes index.
    1. Ovaries — Cancer. I. Title. II. Series.
[DNLM: 1. Ovarian neoplasms.   WP 322 P6930]
RC280.08P58   616.99'465   82-4364
                                 AACR2

Printed in Singapore by Selector Printing Co Pte Ltd

Ovarian Malignancies:
The Clinical Care of Adults and Adolescents

CURRENT REVIEWS IN OBSTETRICS AND GYNAECOLOGY

OBSTETRICS

Series Editor

Tom Lind MB BS DSc PhD MRCPath MRCOG
MRC Human Reproduction Group, Princess Mary Maternity Hospital, Newcastle upon Tyne

Volumes published
Obstetric Analgesia and Anaesthesia *J. Selwyn Crawford*
Early Diagnosis of Fetal Defects *D.J.H. Brock*
Early Teenage Pregnancy *J.K. Russell*

Volumes in preparation
Coagulation Problems in Pregnancy *E.A. Letsky*
Drugs in Pregnancy *B. Krauer, F. Krauer and F. Hytten*
Immunology of Pregnancy *W. Page Faulk and H. Fox*
Hypertension and Related Problems in Pregnancy *W.A.W. Walters*
Ultrasound in Obstetrics *W.J. Garrett and P.S. Warren*
Fetoscopy *C.H. Rodeck*

GYNAECOLOGY

Series Editors

Albert Singer DPhil PhD FRCOG
Whittington Hospital, London

Joe A. Jordan MD DObst FRCOG
Birmingham Maternity Hospital, Queen Elizabeth Medical Centre, Birmingham

Volumes in preparation

Therapeutic Abortion *A.A. Calder*
Male Infertility *A.M. Jequier*
Cancer of the Cervix *H.M. Shingleton and J. Orr*
Gynaecological Premalignant Disease *A. Singer, F. Sharp and J. Jordan*
The Menopause *M. Thom*
Urinary Incontinence *S.L. R. Stanton, L. Cardozo and P. Hilton*

Foreword

It seems fitting that the first gynaecological text in the *Current Reviews in Obstetrics & Gynaecology Series* should concern itself with the subject of ovarian carcinoma. Of all the major problems confronting the gynaecologist, the management of this malignancy seems to be the most intractable and challenging. That Professor Piver should be invited to edit this first volume is also most appropriate as he has distinguished himself as a basic scientist, clinician and surgeon in the field of ovarian carcinoma. His all-round knowledge of the subject means that a high uniform standard is maintained in all the chapters dealing with the various aspects of diagnosis and treatment.

There are two main objects of this new series. Firstly, to present an up-to-date objective and comprehensive monograph review of important subjects in gynaecology which are directed at the gynaecologist in training and the practising clinician who desires to be brought up-to-date and kept informed on the latest developments in the discipline. The second aim is to have this monograph produced by one or at the most two authors. This means that a certain uniformity and an individual philosophy can be developed throughout the text; something that is impossible to achieve with a multi-authored monograph. Professor Piver, with the help of Professor Robert Scully of Boston who has contributed the chapter on pathology, has achieved both these objectives in this first volume. In following monographs the remaining genital cancers will be reviewed as will other relevant and topical subjects such as infertility, urinary incontinence and pelvic inflammatory disease. Authors have been invited from both the new and old world and this it is hoped will provide a 'fusion of ideas' that will be of benefit to gynaecologists worldwide.

London   Albert Singer
Birmingham   Joseph Jordan
1983

Preface

This book is dedicated to the practising gynaecologists, surgeons and generalists who frequently have the prime responsibility of caring for numerous patients with various illnesses. In doing so, no one physician can be expert in all aspects of diseases of women, but must still have sufficient clinical information to deliver the best health care to the individual patient.

This book will deal, as the title implies, with the clinical care of women with ovarian cancer. Since not all women with ovarian cancer are cured of their disease, many of these concepts will change with time, and many are based on the experience and opinion of the author — both requiring subsequent revision with time and reflection. Notwithstanding these shortcomings, this book is written for the express purpose of aiding the practising physician in the clinical care of patients with ovarian cancer.

Ultimately, any significant improvement in the survival of patients with ovarian cancer will rest on discovering the cause of ovarian cancer and improving methods which will make the diagnosis of ovarian cancer possible in its earliest stages. These two issues, both still unresolved, are dealt with in the opening chapter. The remainder of the book deals with 29 separate ovarian malignancies and the clinical management relative to each individual tumour.

Finally, very special thanks and appreciation to Denise Kendall for her incalculable hours at the typewriter, to Kevin Craig for his excellent suggestions in syntax and vocabulary, to Sylvia Hull for her many letters from the editorial office in England, to Dr Gerald P. Murphy for his continued support in this project, and

Dr Robert E. Scully for adding his very considerable experience and expertise in the pathology of ovarian tumours to this book.

Buffalo, 1983   M.S.P.

Contents

1. *Aetiology and early diagnosis of ovarian cancer*   1
2. *Pathology of ovarian malignancies* Robert E. Scully   19
3. *Borderline ovarian carcinomas*   68
4. *Staging laparotomy in stage I & II ovarian malignancies*   74
5. *The treatment of stage I & II ovarian carcinomas*   83
   Radioactive chromic phosphate (^{32}P)
   Radioactive gold (^{198}Au), Whole abdominal
   irradiation and systemic chemotherapy
6. *First line chemotherapy and debulking surgery for stage III & IV ovarian adenocarcinoma*   99
7. *Second and third-line chemotherapy in metastatic ovarian adenocarcinoma*   110
8. *Second-look laparotomy and second-look laparoscopy in ovarian carcinoma*   116
9. *Brenner tumours of the ovary*   122
10. *Immature ovarian teratomas*   128
11. *Endodermal sinus tumour and embryonal carcinoma of the ovary*   135
12. *Dysgerminoma*   145
13. *Ovarian choriocarcinoma and mixed germ-cell ovarian tumours*   153
14. *Primary ovarian carcinoids*   159
    Insular carcinoid, Trabecular carcinoid, Strumal carcinoid, and Struma ovarii
15. *Granulosa cell tumours*   167
    Granulosa theca cell, Cystic variety of granulosa cell tumours, Juvenile granulosa-theca cell tumours, Thecomas, Sclerosing ovarian stromal tumour, Sex cord tumour with annular tubules (SCTAT), Gynandroblastoma

Contents

16. *Sertoli Leydig and lipid cell tumours of the ovary* 182
Sertoli Leydig cell tumours, Pure Sertoli cell tumour, Lipid cell
tumours, Hilus cell tumours, Stromal Leydig cell tumours

17. *Ovarian sarcomas* 194

Index 201

To Susan, Debra,
Bobbie and Kenny who
are my *raison d'être*.

M.S.P.

Aetiology and early diagnosis of ovarian cancer

Aetiology

Ovarian cancer is a disease of middle and upper class women (Cohort 1955) which occurs primarily in the highly industrialised countries of the world. Some confirmation of this fact is seen in that the highest incidence of ovarian cancer occurs among women in the affluent industrialised countries: Sweden 21/100 000, Norway 16/100 000, United States (white) 15/100 000, England 14/100 000, Israel 11/100 000, United States (black) 5/100 000, Africa 4/100 000, India 3/100 000 and Japan 3/100 000 (Kolstad & Beecham 1975). The major exception to this high geographic incidence is the low rate in highly industrialised Japan. Japanese women, however, who immigrate to the United States, and subsequently, their daughters, have an incidence of ovarian cancer similar to women in the United States.

This geographic prevalence points to a possible causal relationship of one or more industrial chemicals in the development of ovarian cancer. The two industrial chemical products most often implicated are asbestos and talc. Asbestos is implicated because: (1) it has been demonstrated that asbestos is a cause of peritoneal mesotheliomas (Keal 1960), a tumour similar in clinical behaviour and histological appearance to ovarian adenocarcinoma; (2) at least one study has demonstrated an increased incidence of ovarian cancer in women exposed to industrial asbestos (Keal 1960); and (3) injection of asbestos into the peritoneal cavity of rabbits and guinea pigs produces atypical ovarian hyperplasia considered to be consistent with the histological changes seen in early ovarian malignancies (Graham & Graham 1967).

Talc is implicated because of its relationship to asbestos (Longo

& Young 1979). Talc particles are physically similar to asbestos, and until recently, most talc powders contained asbestos. Talc is found in soaps, powders, deodorants, condoms and contraceptive diaphragms. Also, many contraceptive diaphragms and condoms were previously stored in talc powder. The theory is that talc particles migrate to the ovary through the cervix, endometrium and fallopian tubes, with a resultant abnormal proliferation (Fig. 1.1). In at least one study, imbedded talc particles were found in 75% of the ovarian tumours studied (Henderson et al 1971).

Pregnancy, on the other hand, has been suggested as having a protective effect against the development of ovarian cancer. From 1957–1965, over 400 ovarian cancer cases were seen at Roswell Park Memorial Institute. During this period, a detailed questionnaire was completed by all ovarian cancer patients and their age matched controls (Joly et al 1974). The study demonstrated an increased relative risk of ovarian cancer as the total number of pregnancies decreased, and that ovarian cancer patients had the following characteristics: (1) a lower mean number of pregnancies, (2) a larger proportion never pregnant, (3) a larger proportion nulliparous, (4) a later age at first pregnancy, (5) a larger proportion who tried and failed to become pregnant; and (6) an increased frequency of miscarriages compared to the controls. This protective effect of pregnancy has been documented by others (Beral et al 1978), although the mechanism remains speculative. Confir-

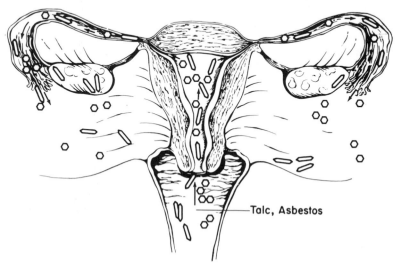

Fig. 1.1 Possible mechanism by which talc or asbestos particles reach the ovary

mation of this is also seen in the fact that ovarian cancer is rare in populations where birth control is not practised. The present increase in the use of oral contraceptives, intrauterine devices, and the increased number of abortions being performed may be possible causes for the increased incidence of ovarian cancer which has been observed during the past two decades.

To date, there has been no documented association between oral contraceptives and the development of ovarian cancer. There have been reports, however, on the relationship of breast and endometrial carcinoma to ovarian cancer, thereby implicating hormones as being possibly related to the aetiology of ovarian cancer. Confirmation of the relationship of these three hormonally-dependent areas is seen in that women with breast carcinoma have twice the standard risk of developing ovarian cancer, and that a similar, but lower, risk occurs in women with endometrial carcinoma (Wynder et al 1969 Shoffenfeld & Berg 1971).

No viral aetiology has been suggested as a possible cause in the development of ovarian cancer. Conversely, however, several, but not all, studies have demonstrated a lower incidence of a history of mumps in ovarian cancer patients, compared to controls. This fact postulates a possible protective effect of mumps oophoritis in relationship to the lower incidence of ovarian cancer in such patients (West 1966).

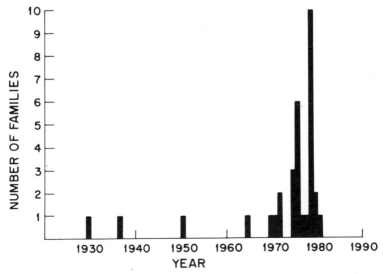

Fig. 1.2 Number of case reports of families with ovarian cancer per year since 1929. Reprinted by permission of Obstetrics and Gynecology

3

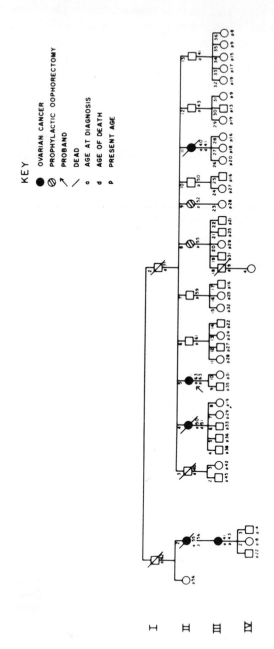

Fig. 1.3 Pedigree of family with ovarian carcinoma. Reprinted by permission of Obstetrics and Gynecology

4

In certain women, there appears to be an hereditary (familial) factor in the development of ovarian cancer. The type of transmission appears to be autosomal dominant in most instances. For some inexplicable reason, there has been an increase in the number of reports of familial ovarian cancer in the past 10 years, especially as compared to the dearth of such reports prior to 1970 (Fig. 1.2). At Roswell Park Memorial Institute, two families with familial ovarian cancer were seen, each having five family members with ovarian carcinoma. The first pedigree consisted of the mother, three daughters and grandaughters ovarian cancer (Lurain & Piver 1979). The pedigree of the second family is presented in Fig. 1.3 and consisted of three sisters, a first cousin and her daughter (Piver et al 1981). If an autosomal dominant transmission is eventually established as the mode of transmission in instances of familial ovarian cancer, genetic counselling for prophylactic oophorectomy, at an appropriate age, may lead to a decrease in deaths from ovarian cancer in such families.

Early diagnosis

Although there has been significant progress in improved surgical staging for presumed localised ovarian carcinoma (stage I and II), and improved debulking surgery and more effective combination chemotherapy in advanced (stages III and IV) ovarian cancer patients, significant improvement in the overall five-year survival rate will not be achieved until tests for early detection can be devised (Table 1.1). Although ovarian cancer ranks third in incidence behind cervical and endometrial malignancies, respectively, it is the leading cause of death from gynaecologic malignancies. It is the disease that eventually will occur in 1.4% of all new born females. Moreover, two-thirds of all women with ovarian cancer will die from the malignancy. Even with the significant improvements in surgery, radiotherapy and chemotherapy, the death rate has not significantly changed in the past 20 years. Significant in this high mortality rate is the fact that ovarian cancer is a 'hidden' cancer that is not easily detected by physical or laboratory examination, and that is not associated with significant symptomatology in the early stages of the disease. Therefore, 70% of women have metastasis beyond the pelvis (stage III and IV) at the initial diagnosis.

Earlier detection and diagnosis of ovarian cancer will come

5

Table 1.1 FIGO staging: carcinoma of the ovary. International Federation Gynaecologists and Obstetricians

Stage I:	Growth limited to the ovaries
IA:	Growth limited to one ovary; no ascites 1. No tumour on the external surface; capsule intact 2. Tumour present on the external surface and/or capsule ruptured
IB:	Growth limited to both ovaries; no ascites 1. No tumour on the external surface; capsule intact 2. Tumour present on the external surface and/or capsule ruptured
IC:	Tumour either stage IA or IB, but with ascites* present or positive peritoneal washings
Stage II:	Growth involving one or both ovaries with pelvic extension
IIA:	Extension and/or metastases to the uterus and/or tubes
IIB:	Extension to other pelvic tissues
IIC:	Tumour either stage IIA or IIB, but with ascites* present or positive peritoneal washings
Stage III:	Growth involving one or both ovaries with intraperitoneal metastases outside the pelvis and/or positive retroperitoneal nodes Tumour limited to the true pelvis with histologically proven malignant extension to small bowel or omentum
Stage IV:	Growth involving one or both ovaries with distant metastases. If pleural effusion is present there must be positive cytology to allot a case to stage IV Parenchymal liver metastases equals stage IV
Special category:	Unexplored cases which are thought to be ovarian carcinoma

* Ascites is peritoneal effusion which in the opinion of the surgeon is pathologic and/or clearly exceeds normal amounts

about when: (1) physicians have a higher degree of suspicion, especially in middle and upper class women with vague pelvic and abdominal symptoms; (2) pelvic examination becomes a routine part of the physical examination; and (3) a serum immunological test, specific for early stage ovarian cancer, is developed.

Symptomatology in ovarian cancer patients

The most common symptoms of ovarian cancer are abdominal pain, increasing abdominal girth, bloating, non-specific digestive abnormalities, pelvic 'discomfort,' and abnormal uterine (vaginal) bleeding. Of 100 consecutive ovarian cancer patients referred to Roswell Park Memorial Institute during 1971–1972 (Table 1.2), abdominal distension was the most common presenting symptom

Table 1.2 Initial symptom in 100 patients with ovarian cancer treated during 1971–1972 (Piver et al 1976)

Symptoms	Number of patients
Abdominal distension	44
Lower abdominal pain	33
Pelvic mass on routine examination*	15
Vaginal bleeding	13
Abdominal mass	9
Weight loss	4
Dyspnoea or chest pain	3
Gall bladder colic	2
Pelvic inflammatory disease	1
Vomiting	1
Abnormal pap smear	1
Supraclavicular mass	1
Breast mass	1
Fractured wrist	1

* Asymptomatic (15%)

(44%) followed by lower abdominal pain (33%), and abnormal uterine (vaginal) bleeding (13%) (Piver et al 1976).

Pelvic examination in the early diagnosis of ovarian cancer

Although it has been estimated that only 1 in 10 000 ovarian cancers will be detected by routine pelvic examination, a review of 100 consecutive ovarian cancer patients seen at Roswell Park Memorial Institute documented that 15% were diagnosed in this manner (Piver et al 1976). Some investigators have also advocated using culdocenteses, whereby saline is injected through the vagina into the cul-de-sac, aspirated and examined cytologically (Funkhouser et al 1975). Unfortunately, this procedure has not proven to be effective in early ovarian cancer detection, and it is not acceptable to patients.

Preliminary suspicions of an ovarian malignancy are still confirmed by pelvic examination. The smallest ovarian mass that could be diagnosed by this means would be 1 cm^3 in diameter, weighing 1 gram, and containing one billion cancer cells. Palpation of a 1 cm^3 ovarian tumour remains, at best, difficult; and, at worst, nearly impossible. However, 95% of ovarian cancers measure more than 5 cm in diameter. Therefore, the finding of a 5 cm or larger ovarian mass on pelvic examination, especially in a 40 to 60 year-old patient, requires further evaluation to determine ovarian malignancy. An exception to this dictum would be a 5 cm cystic mass in a young menstruating female. The cyst may be functional and not malignant, and should be treated by observation and/or hormonal therapy. However, if it does not regress within a two-month period of treatment, it should be suspected as being an ovarian malignancy. Since 25% of ovarian cancers are bilateral at initial presentation, in contrast to 5% for benign ovarian tumours, the finding of a bilateral ovarian tumour on pelvic examination requires immediate evaluation for ovarian malignancy.

Ultrasonography, computerised tomography and laparoscopy in the diagnosis of ovarian cancer

It is important to determine if a pelvic mass is a benign uterine leiomyoma, an inflammatory condition of the fallopian tubes or ovaries, a benign ovarian cyst, a bowel tumour, or an ovarian malignancy, all of which require different therapies.

Ultrasonography, computerised axial tomography (CAT), and laparoscopy offer alternative methods to formal laparotomy for diagnosing suspicious pelvic masses that are discovered by pelvic examination. Neither ultrasonography or a CAT scan can distinguish a benign from a malignant ovarian tumour. However, abnormal areas of increased echo production on ultrasound may suggest ovarian cancer.

The value of CAT scan in the early diagnosis of ovarian cancer has not been established. The drawbacks are the radiation exposure, the lack of clarity of detail in very obese or extremely thin patients, and the small risk of reaction to the contrast media. The advantages of ultrasound are that there is no radiation exposure, there is no possibility for reaction to contrast media, and that it is superior to CAT scan in differentiating cystic from the more frequently malignant solid ovarian tumours. Ultrasonography is 80 to 90% accurate in diagnosing size, location and consistency of ovarian tumours, and in separating ovarian tumours from benign uterine leiomyoma. The disadvantages of ultrasound are in detecting masses that are 2 cm or less in diameter, and in differentiating intestinal loops of bowel, pelvic inflammatory disease, ectopic pregnancy and pelvic endometriosis from an ovarian tumour.

Laparoscopy is an important alternative to formal laparotomy in distinguishing benign uterine leiomyoma and benign ovarian pathology from ovarian cancer. This was demonstrated by Samuelsson & Sjovall (1970) who performed laparoscopies on 83 patients who had a preoperative clinical diagnosis of benign uterine leiomyoma. Their study showed that only 66% had leiomyoma, whereas 12% had associated fallopian tube and ovarian pathology and 22% had only fallopian tube and ovarian disease. Similarly, Frangenheim & Stockhammer (1969) demonstrated the value of laparoscopy in preventing a laparotomy in a significant number of patients with pelvic masses. They performed diagnostic laparoscopy on 218 postmenopausal women with pelvic masses. Malignant disease was present in 42 (19.7%): 19 had ovarian cancer, 14 had intestinal cancers, and 9 had malignant metastatic ovarian lesions. Laparotomy for benign disease was unnecessary in 60.4% of their patients.

Preoperative evaluation

Once an ovarian malignancy is suspected either by pelvic examination, ultrasonography, CAT scan or laparoscopy, the following tests are of value prior to formal laparotomy: barium enema, upper gastrointestinal radiological examination, intravenous pyelogram, chest X-ray, lymphangiography, and serum tests of liver function (Table 1.3).

Table 1.3 Preoperative evaluation in ovarian cancer

Examination	Value
Barium enema	Colon cancer metastatic to the ovary
Upper gastrointestinal series	Gastric cancer metastatic to the ovary
Intravenous pyelography	Ureteral involvement: pelvic kidney
Lymphangiography	Pelvic & para-aortic nodal metastasis
Serum tests of liver function	Liver metastasis
Chest X-ray	Diaphragmatic or pulmonary metastasis

Barium enema should be performed because of the high frequency with which rectosigmoid carcinomas metastasise to the ovary. Upper gastrointestinal radiological examination is of value because gastric carcinomas and other gastrointestinal tumours frequently metastasise to both ovaries (Krukenberg tumour). Preoperative chest X-ray may demonstrate an elevation of the right leaf of the diaphragm or a right pleural effusion that is secondary to the frequent occurrence of metastasis to the right leaf of the diaphragm, even from stage I ovarian malignancies. An intravenous pyelogram is of value in ruling out the rare occurrence of a pelvic kidney as the cause of the pelvic mass, and to evaluate ureteral involvement by an ovarian tumour. Liver function tests may be abnormal and may indicate liver metastasis. Since retroperitoneal lymph node metastasis occurs in at least 10% of even stage I ovarian cancer patients, preoperative bipedal lymphangiography may be helpful in locating such metastasis at the time of laparotomy.

Immunodiagnosis of ovarian cancer

Due to the lack of symptoms in early stages of ovarian cancer, improving early diagnosis must depend on the development of a serum test that is specific for ovarian cancer. For a serum test to be useful, the substance would have to be produced by the ovarian tumour in its earliest growth phase and in sufficient quantities to be easily measurable. An ideal serum marker would also decrease with successful treatment, increase with early recurrence and quantitatively correlate with the amount of tumour present.

The development of such a site specific marker is possible because in the conversion from normality to malignancy, cells develop molecular markers that occur primarily on the cell membrane and that allow for the designation of the cancer cells by immunological means. These molecular markers on the cell membrane are primarily glycoproteins, many of which are antigens that are capable of eliciting an immune response in the host leading to production of specific antibodies.

Detection of these antigens in serum is possible because they are released into the circulation either (1) during the time of cell death or lysis, (2) by abnormal permeability of the cell membrane, or (3) by normal divestment of the cell membrane into the circulation.

At present, it is possible to measure a significant number of tumour markers in the serum of ovarian cancer patients. Although the development of such tumour markers is essential for early diagnosis, none has been found to be elevated in the majority of patients with early stage ovarian cancer — a requisite for their value in screening asymptomatic women.

In general, the substances are categorised as (1) carcinoplacental antigens, (2) fetal antigens, (3) tumour-associated antigens, and (4) miscellaneous tumour markers. Some of these tumour

Table 1.4 Immunodiagnosis of ovarian cancer

Carcinoplacental antigens	Fetal antigens	Tumour associated antigens	Miscellaneous
Regan isoenzyme	Carcinoembryonic antigen	OCAA*	Fibrin degradation products
Nagao isoenzyme	Alpha-fetoprotein	OCA†	Galactosyltransferase
Bjorklund isoenzyme	Beta-oncofetal protein		Alpha-L-fucosidase
Human chorionic gonadotrophin	Fetal ferritin		
Human placental lactogen			
Pregnancy specific glycoprotein			

* Ovarian cystadenocarcinoma associated antigen
† Ovarian cancer antigen

markers are found only in epithelial ovarian cancers, whereas others are specific for ovarian germ-cell tumours (Table 1.4).

I. Carcinoplacental antigens

The ectopically produced carcinoplacental antigens which are normally present only in the placenta include placental alkaline phosphatases (Regan isoenzyme, Nagao isoenzyme and Bjorklund isoenzyme), and placental hormones (human chorionic gonadotrophin, human placental lactogen and pregnancy specific glycoprotein SP_1).

a. Placental alkaline phosphatases

The placental alkaline phosphatases are biochemically distinct from those found in the bone, liver, kidney and intestine. After malignant transformation of certain tissues, they are ectopically produced in ovarian, lung, breast and gastric carcinomas.

(i) Regan isoenzyme

The Regan isoenzyme is elevated in most patients with ovarian cancer, and to a lesser degree, in many other malignancies (Cadeau et al 1974).

11

(ii) Nagao Isoenzyme

The Nagao isoenzyme is the delta phenotype of the Regan isoenzyme. It has been reported to be elevated in over 70% of ovarian cancer patients, but it is also elevated in 35% of non-ovarian cancer patients (Inglis et al 1973).

(iii) Bjorklund Isoenzyme

The Bjorklund isoenzyme has been isolated from the human placenta. It has been reported to be elevated in 50% of ovarian cancer patients, but it is also elevated in many other malignancies (Bjorklund 1972).

Placental hormones

(i) Human chorionic gonadotrophin (HCG)

HCG is normally elevated only during pregnancy and, therefore, its detection at other times implies ectopic production by a tumour. It is elevated in as many as 41% of all ovarian cancer patients (Samaan et al 1976); but it is elevated in over 90% of patients with specific ovarian germ-cell tumours: embryonal carcinoma, ovarian choriocarcinoma and ovarian teratomas admixed with embryonal carcinoma or choriocarcinoma.

(ii) Human placental lactogen (HPL)

HPL has been reported to be elevated in as many as 76% of patients with common epithelial ovarian tumours (Samaan et al 1976); but it is more specific for germ-cell ovarian tumours containing ectopic trophoblastic tissue.

(iii) Pregnancy specific glycoprotein (SP_1)

SP_1 is elevated in a significant number of ovarian germ-cell tumours containing trophoblastic tissue (Bagshawe et al 1980). The value of SP_1 in detecting ovarian germ-cell tumours is negated by the extreme sensitivity of HCG in detecting much smaller volumes of residual tumour than SP_1. Pregnancy-associated proteins have also been demonstrated in breast, bowel and other malignancies.

II. Fetal antigens

Fetal antigens are primarily glycoproteins that are present in the fetus during the first and second trimesters, and that disappear after birth. With the development of certain malignancies, they reappear on the cancer cell surface membrane. Included in this category are carcinoembryonic antigen (CEA), alpha-fetoprotein (AFP), beta-oncofetoprotein (BOFA), and fetal ferritin. Unlike tumour-associated antigens, they are minimally antigenic, they may occur in various tumours and normal tissues, and they are cross reactive with other tumours.

a. Carcinoembryonic antigen (CEA)

CEA is normally present in the embryonic intestine during the first and second trimesters, and is normally absent at birth. Although elevated in as many as 77% of various cancer patients, it is also elevated in cervical (67%) and endometrial (59%) carcinomas, as well as vulvar, lung, bladder and breast cancer, and most commonly, in colon carcinoma (Khoo & Mackay 1974). Also, low-level elevations are present in non-malignant diseases such as chronic lung disease, secondary to smoking, and chronic inflammatory bowel disease. CEA is elevated in 26–48% of stage I ovarian malignancies and in relatively higher percentages of stages II, III, and IV (Table 1.5) (DiSaia et al 1975, van Nagell et al 1975).

Table 1.5 Incidence of elevated CEA levels in ovarian cystadenocarcinoma

Stage	DiSaia et al 1975	Khoo & Mackay 1974	van Nagell et al 1975
I	26%	48%	42%
II	50%	50%	33%
III	58%	78%	32%
IV	73%	90%	56%

b. Alpha-fetoprotein (AFP)

AFP is a fetal antigen produced in the human liver and yolk sac of the placenta in the first two trimesters, and is not normally present at birth. It is a specific tumour marker for endodermal sinus tumour of the ovary, embryonal carcinoma of the ovary, and ovarian teratomas admixed with either of these tumours. It is not elevated in epithelial ovarian carcinomas. It is elevated in most patients with endodermal sinus tumour of the ovary, decreases with response to therapy and increases with recurrence, making it almost a perfect tumour marker for this disease (Sell et al 1976).

c. Beta-oncofetoprotein (BOFA)

BOFA is elevated in ovarian cancer patients, but it is not specific for ovarian cancer (Fritsch & Mach 1975).

d. Fetal ferritin

Similarly, fetal ferritin has been elevated in ovarian cancer patients, but it is not specific for ovarian cancer (Alpert et al 1973).

III. Tumour-associated antigens

Tumour-associated antigens are glycoproteins that are present on the cell surface of ovarian cancer cells, but that have not been shown to be present in the non-malignant ovarian epithelial cells from which they were derived. It is theorised that these ovarian cancer tumour-associated antigens are acquired during the malignant transformation process. What causes the alteration in the host's DNA which results in these glycoproteins is not known. However, these glycoproteins can elicit an immune response in the majority of patients with epithelial ovarian carcinomas.

Glycoproteins have been demonstrated to be immunologically distinct from carcinoembryonic antigens, alpha-fetaprotein, blood group substances, and normal histocompatible antigens, and are not found in normal ovarian tissues, benign cystadenomas or other ovarian malignancies.

The ovarian cancer associated antigens were first demonstrated when an antitumour antiserum (antibody) in rabbits was developed against extracts of surgical specimens of human ovarian cystadenocarcinomas. Using immunodiffusion experiments, the antigens specific for cystadenocarcinoma were found not to cross react with other malignant tissues. Immunodiffusion experiments showed a major line of identity (antigen-antibody precipitin) forming between the cystadenocarcinomas and the antitumour serum, but not between the sera of other malignancies.

The detection of low levels (nanograms/millilitre) of ovarian carcinoma associated antigen requires the development of a specific radioimmune assay (RIA) for the detection of the antigen in serum. Serum of a patient suspected of having ovarian cancer is exposed to antibodies (raised in rabbits) against the ovarian tumour antigen. The radiolabelled ovarian tumour antigen is then added to compete for binding sites with unlabelled ovarian cancer antigen in the patient's serum. The higher the patient's ovarian cancer antigen concentration, the smaller the amount of radiolabelled ovarian cancer antigen bound. A decrease in the binding activity in the serum gives a measurement by radioimmune assay of the amount of ovarian cancer.

Knauf & Urbach (1980) have demonstrated an ovarian tumour-associated antigen, referred to as OCA, in the plasma of ovarian cancer patients. Of 153 patients with ovarian cancer, 76% had elevated OCA levels. Why OCA was not detected in all ovarian cancer patients, or elevated in a significantly higher percentage of more advanced staged patients, remains a major question and a significant shortcoming to its value as a screening test (Table 1.6).

Table 1.6 Plasma OCA levels: Knauff & Urbach (1980)

Stage	Patients	% positive OCA
I	27	78
II	54	74
III	57	79
IV	15	67
Total	153	76

Barlow & Bhattacharya (1979) found an ovarian cancer associated antigen, OCAA (ovarian cystadenocarcinoma associated antigen), which was elevated in 70% of stage III and IV ovarian cancer patients. Using radioimmune assays for OCAA in 60 women with ovarian adenocarcinoma, elevated levels were present in stage II, III and IV patients (Table 1.7). Also, 16 women who had elevated OCAA levels before resection of malignant ovarian masses, showed a drop in serum OCAA levels two to three weeks after surgery. However, the correlation between the clinical course and the fall and rise of OCAA occurred in only 70% of the patients followed serially.

Table 1.7 Concentration of circulating ovarian cystadenocarcinoma associated antigen in the sera of ovarian cancer patients (Piver et al 1979)

Stage	Patients	OCAA 10 ng/ml	%
I	1	0	0
II	3	2	66.6
III	41	27	65.8
IV	15	12	80.0

IV. Miscellaneous tumour markers

a. Fibrin degradation products (FDP)

It has been postulated that there is an increased fibrinolytic activity associated with ovarian cancer that results in increased levels of fibrin degradation products (fibrin-fibrinogen) in the sera of ovarian cancer patients. Increased FDP levels indicate that fibrinolysis has occurred, but does not signify the presence of disseminated intravascular coagulation. In one report, FDP levels were elevated in 94% (16/17) of the ovarian cancer patients studied (Anstey & Blythe 1978). However, since FDP is elevated in numerous benign and malignant conditions, it is not a useful screening test for early ovarian cancer detection.

b. Galactosyltransferase

Galactosyltransferase, a glycoprotein, has been elevated in most ovarian cancer patients (Bhattacharya & Barlow 1979). To date, however, it has not been tested or evaluated in early stage ovarian cancer, and it is also elevated in other malignancies.

c. Alpha-L-fucosidase

Alpha-L-fucosidase is the only serum enzyme studied to date that may be a specific genetic marker for ovarian carcinoma patients. It was demonstrated to be significantly *deficient* in the serum of patients with ovarian carcinoma compared to other tumours (Bhattacharya & Barlow 1979). If further elaboration of this study corroborates this finding, this could be the ideal tumour marker for detecting early ovarian cancer in susceptible patients.

Aetiology and early diagnosis of ovarian cancer

The diagnostic value of ovarian cancer associated antigens and other similar molecular tumour markers will be confirmed only if they can be detected in the sera of asymptomatic women who subsequently are found to have early ovarian cancer; and if, on purification of the antigen and further testing, they more consistently correlate with response to therapy. Purification of these substances and further characterisation should lead to a specific immunological screening test for the early detection of ovarian cancer and thus subsequently lead to improved survival for women with ovarian cancer.

REFERENCES

Alpert E R, Coston R L, Drysdale J W 1973 Carcino-fetal human liver ferritins. Nature 242: 194
Anstey J T, Blythe J G 1978 Fibrin degradation products and the diagnosis of ovarian carcinoma. Obstetrics & Gynecology 52: 605 608
Bagshawe K D, Wass M, Searle F 1980 Markers in gynecologic cancer. Archives Gynecology 229: 303
Beral V, Fraser P, Chilvers C 1978 Does pregnancy protect against ovarian cancer? Lancet: 1083–1087
Bhattacharya M, Barlow J J 1979 Tumour markers for ovarian cancer. International Advances in Surgical Oncology 2: 155–176
Bjorklund B 1972 Immunological techniques for the detection of cancer. In Bjorklund B (ed): Proceedings of the Folksam Symposium. Bonniers, Stockholm, Sweden
Cadeau B J, Blakstein M E, Malkin A 1974 Increased incidence of placental-like alkaline phosphatase activity in breast and genitourinary cancer. Cancer Research 34: 729
Cohort E U 1955 Socio-economic distribution of cancer of female sex organ in New Haven. Cancer 8: 3
DiSaia P J, Haverback B J, Dyce B J, Morrow C P 1975 Carcinoembryonic antigen in patients with gynecologic malignancies. American Journal of Obstetrics & Gynecology 121: 159–172
Fritsch R, Mach J P 1975 Identification of a new oncofetal antigen associated with several types of human carcinomas. Nature 258: 734
Frangenheim H, Stockhammer H 1969 La laparoscopie dans le diagnostic-differentie des tumeurs du petit bassin chez les femmes menopausées. Gynaecologia (Basel) 167: 503
Funkhouser J W, Hunter K K Thompson N J 1975 The diagnostic value of cul-de-sac aspiration on the detection of ovarian carcinoma. Acta cytologyica 19: 538–541
Graham J, Graham R 1967 Ovarian cancer and asbestos. Environmental Research 1: 115
Henderson W J, Joslin C A F, Turnbull A C, Griffiths K 1971 Talc and carcinoma of the ovary and cervix. Obstetrics & Gynecology Breast Commission 78: 266
Inglis N R, Kirley S, Stolbach L L, et al 1973 Phenotypes of the Regan isoenzyme and idemnity between the placental D-variant and Nagao isoenzyme. Cancer Research 33: 1657.

Joly, D J, Lilienfeld A M, Diamond E B, Bross I D 1974 An epidemiologic study of the relationship of reproductive experience to cancer of the ovary. American Journal of Epidemiology 99: 190–209

Keal E E December 3, 1960 Asbestosis and abdominal neoplasms. Lancet: 1211–1216

Khoo S K, Mackay E V 1974 Carcinoembryonic antigen by radioimmunoassay in the detection of recurrence during long-term follow-up of female genital cancer. Cancer 34: 542–548

Knauf S, Urbach G I 1980 A study of ovarian cancer patients using a radioimmunoassay for human ovarian tumour-associated antigen OCA. American Journal of Obstetrics & Gynecology 138: 1222–1223

Kolstad P, Beecham J C 1975 Epidemiology of ovarian neoplasia. Congressional Serial Number 364: 56, 964

Longo D L, Young R C August 18, 1979 Cosmetic talc and ovarian cancer. Lancet 349–351

Lurain J R, Piver M S 1979 Familial ovarian cancer. Gynecologic Oncology 8: 185

van Nagell J R, Meeker W R, Parker J C, Harralson J D 1975 Carcino-embryonic antigen in patients with gynecologic malignancy. Cancer 35: 1372–1376

Piver M S, Barlow J J, Bhattacharya M 1979 Treatment and immunodiagnosis of advanced ovarian adenocarcinoma: a preliminary report. Cancer Treatment Reports 63: 265–267

Piver M S, S, Barlow J J, Sawyer D 1981 Familial ovarian cancer: Increasing in frequency. Obstetrics & Gynecology (in press)

Piver M S, Lele S B, Barlow J J 1976 Preoperative and intraoperative evaluation in ovarian malignancy. Obstetrics & Gynecology 48: 312–315

Samaan N A, Smith J P, Rutledge F N, Schultz P N 1976 The significance of measurement of human placental lactogen, human chorionic gonadotropin and carcinoembryonic antigen in patients with ovarian carcinoma. American Journal of Obstetrics & Gynecology 126: 186–188

Samuelsson S, Sjovall A 1970 The value of laparoscopy in the differential diagnosis between uterine fibromyomata and adnexal tumours. Acta obstetrica et cytologica scandanavica 49: 175

Sell A, Sogaad H, Nargaad-Pederson B 1976 Serum alfa-fetoprotein as a marker for the effect of postoperative radiation therapy and/or chemotherapy in 8 cases. International Journal of Cancer 18: 574

Shoffenfeld D, Berg J 1971 Incidence of multiple primary cancers. XIV. Cancers of the Female Breast and Genital Organs 46: 161

West R O 1966 Epidemiologic study of malignancies of the ovaries. Cancer 19: 1001

Wynder E L, Dodo H, Barber H R 1969 Epidemiology of cancer of the ovary. Cancer 23: 352

18

2

Pathology of ovarian malignancies

Introduction

Knowledge of the pathology of ovarian tumours is essential to understanding their behaviour and selecting the optimal therapy. The ovary is the site of a wider variety of tumours than any other organ, and the oft-repeated precept that ovarian neoplasia is not one but many diseases is fully justified by the range of its biological manifestations (Fox & Langley 1976, Scully 1977a, 1979a). Only within the last two decades, as the result of deliberations by the International Federation of Gynecology and Obstetrics (FIGO) and the World Health Organisation (WHO) committees (Serov & Scully 1972), has a classification with precise definitions of various types of ovarian tumours emerged and become accepted by most investigators. Use of the terminology proposed by these organisations is beginning to result in more meaningful epidemiological and comparative therapeutic data than have been achievable in the past. The WHO classification of ovarian tumours is presented in Table 2.1.

Common epithelial tumours

Common epithelial tumours account for approximately two-thirds of all ovarian neoplasms, and for almost 90% of ovarian cancers in the Western World. Common epithelial tumours are generally considered to be derived from the 'surface epithelium' of the ovary, which descends from the coelomic epithelium, or from the mesothelium of the embryonic gonad. The latter is continuous with the coelomic epithelium which penetrates the underlying mesenchyme to form the Mullerian duct. This proximity is reflected in the various directions of Mullerian differentiation pursued by the surface epithelium when it undergoes neoplasia in the postnatal ovary, i.e., fallopian tube epithelium in cases of serous neoplasia, endometrial epithelium in cases of endometrioid tumours, and endocervical epithelium in cases of mucinous neoplasia.

As a woman approaches menopause, and sometimes earlier in her reproductive life, but rarely before puberty, the surface epithelium extends downward into the ovarian stroma to form surface epithelial inclusion glands, which may become cystic. Although common epithelial tumours may arise from the surface epithelium directly, and grow exophytically, more commonly, they appear to originate from its inclusion glands, accounting for the fact that most of these tumours are basically cystic or endophytic. They are usually solid when they contain a large component of stromal origin or when the neoplastic cells are malignant and proliferate to form masses.

Some common epithelial tumours do not always originate from the surface epithelium, but are designated as common epithelial tumours to avoid confusion. For example the Brenner tumour has been observed to arise in the region of the rete or within a teratoma. Similarly, some mucinous tumours may be monophyletic endodermal teratomas. The evidence suggesting such an interpretation includes the 5% frequency of adjacent dermoid cysts, the common occurrence of mucinous glands in the walls of the dermoid cysts and within other types of teratoma, and the lining of mucinous cystic tumours by intestinal rather than endocervical-type epithelium in at least 25% of the cases. The latter finding, however, does not necessarily indicate an endodermal origin, but may reflect neometaplasia of the surface epithelium in an endodermal direction.

Common epithelial tumours are not always homogeneous and careful study of individual specimens often reveals the presence of two or even three cell types. However, usually no more than a minor component of a second or third cell type is present, and under those circumstances, the neoplasm is classified on the basis of its predominant cellular element.

In addition to being designated according to cell type, common epithelial tumours are subclassified according to three criteria, two architectural and the third involving the degree and character of proliferation of the neoplastic cells. Some tumours, particularly those in the serous category, may be exophytic or cystic, or both. When exophytic growth is present, the word surface is added to the designation. Except for the benign form of Brenner tumour, which characteristically has a predominant stromal component, most common epithelial neoplasms are primarily epithelial, with only a minor portion derived from the ovarian stroma. On the rare occasions when such tumours have a predominant stromal component, the term adenofibroma or cystadenofibroma, modified by the cell type of the neoplasm is used.

A controversial feature of the WHO classification of common epithelial tumours is that neoplasms which are intermediate in their histological features and behaviour, between benign forms and obvious cancers, are included. Although FIGO has preferred the designation carcinoma of low malignant potential for such tumours, the term borderline malignancy was chosen by the WHO. The tumours are characterised by an unusual degree of proliferation of the neoplastic epithelial cells, greater than seen in benign tumours, but a lack of 'destructive' invasion of the stromal component of the neoplasm. Borderline tumours are capable of implanting on the peritoneal surfaces and may be invasive; and in an unknown number of cases, of metastasising to lymph nodes. The diagnosis of borderline malignancy is based, however, on an examination of the primary tumour, without regard for the presence or absence of extension beyond the ovary. The reason for this diagnostic approach is that survival is typically prolonged even in cases in which implantation has taken place. Nevertheless, borderline tumours are truly malignant and may progress to cause the death of the patient, sometimes only after many years. The epithelial proliferation with borderline tumours is characterised by varying degrees of nuclear atypicality and mitotic activity, which are usually minor, stratification of the neoplastic cells, and the formation of cellular buds which appear to be detached from the lining of the cysts of the surface of the tumour.

The subclassification of the common epithelial tumours varies in emphasis from one neoplastic cell type to another. These differences will be mentioned during the following discussions of the individual types.

Serous tumours

Serous tumours are among the most common ovarian tumours.

Table 2.1 Histologic classification of ovarian tumours

Common 'epithelial' tumours
Serous tumours
Benign
Cystadenoma and papillary
cystadenoma
Surface papilloma
Adenofibroma and
cystadenofibroma
Of borderline malignancy
(carcinomas of low malignant
potential)
Cystadenoma and papillary
cystadenoma
Surface papilloma
Adenofibroma and
cystadenofibroma
Malignant
Adenocarcinoma, papillary
adenocarcinoma, and papillary
cystadenocarcinoma
Surface papillary carcinoma
Malignant adenofibroma and
cystadenofibroma

Mucinous tumours
Benign
Cystadenoma
Adenofibroma and
cystadenofibroma
Of borderline malignancy
(carcinomas of low malignant
potential)
Cystadenoma
Adenofibroma and
cystadenofibroma
Malignant
Adenocarcinoma and
cystadenocarcinoma
Malignant adenofibroma and
cystadenofibroma

Endometrioid tumours
Benign
Adenoma and cystadenoma
Adenofibroma and
cystadenofibroma
Of borderline malignancy
(carcinomas of low malignant
potential)
Adenoma and cystadenoma

Adenofibroma and
cystadenofibroma
Malignant
Carcinoma
Adenocarcinoma
Adenoacanthoma
Adenosquamous carcinoma
Malignant adenofibroma and
cystadenofibroma
Endometrioid stromal sarcomas
Mesodermal (mullerian)
adenosarcoma
Mesodermal (mullerian) mixed
tumours, homologous and
heterologous

Clear cell (mesonephroid) tumours
Benign
Adenofibroma
Of borderline malignancy
(carcinomas low malignant
potential)
Malignant
Carcinoma and
adenocarcinoma

Brenner tumours
Benign
of borderline malignancy
(proliferating)
Malignant

Mixed epithelial tumours
Benign
Of borderline malignancy
Malignant

Undifferentiated carcinoma

Unclassified epithelial tumours

Sex cord-stromal tumours
Granulosa-stromal cell tumours
Granulosa cell tumour
Tumours in the thecoma-fibroma
group
Thecoma
Fibroma
Unclassified
Sclerosing stromal tumour
Others

Table 2.1 (Contd).

Sertoli-Leydig cell tumours:
  androblastomas
Well differentiated
  Sertoli cell tumour; tubular
    androblastoma (tubular
    adenoma of Pick)
  Sertoli cell tumour with lipid
    storage; tubular
    androblastoma with lipid
    storage (folliculome lipidique
    of Lecene)
  Sertoli-Leydig cell tumour
    (tubular adenoma with Leydig
    cells)
  Leydig cell tumour; hilus cell
    tumour
    Stromal Leydig cell tumour
  Of intermediate differentiation
  Poorly differentiated (sarcomatoid)
  With heterologous elements

Gynandroblastoma
Unclassified
  Sex cord tumour with annular tubules
  Others

Lipid (Lipoid) cell tumour

Germ cell tumours
  Dysgerminoma
  Endodermal sinus tumour
  Embryonal carcinoma
  Polyembryoma
  Choriocarcinoma
  Teratomas
    Immature
    Mature
      Solid
      Cystic
        Dermoid cyst (mature cystic
          teratoma)
        Dermoid cyst with malignant
          transformation

Monodermal and highly
  specialised
  Struma ovarii
  Carcinoid
  Strumal carcinoid
  Others
Mixed forms

**Mixed germ cell and sex
cord-stromal tumours**

  Gonadoblastoma
    Pure
    Mixed with dysgerminoma or
      other form of germ cell
      tumour
  Others

**Soft tissue tumours not specific to
ovary**

Unclassified tumours

Secondary (metastatic) tumours

Tumour-like conditions
  Pregnancy luteoma
  Hyperplasia of ovarian stroma and
    stromal hyperthecosis
  Massive oedema
  Solitary follicle cyst and corpus
    luteum cyst
  Multiple follicle cysts (polycystic
    ovaries)
  Multiple luteinized follicle cysts
    and/or corpora lutea
    (hyperreactio luteinalis)
  Endometriosis
  Surface-epithelial inclusion cysts
    (germinal inclusion cysts)
  Simple cysts
  Inflammatory lesions
  Parovarian cysts

They are usually cystic, but may be exophytic, or show a combination of cystic and surface growth. Benign and borderline serous cystic tumours typically form unilocular cysts which usually contain serous, but occasionally mucinous, fluid. The benign neoplasms may have uniform, thin flat linings, but sometimes have coarse, hard or soft stromal polypoid excrescences composed mainly of dense or oedematous stroma which protrude into their cavities. The serous borderline tumours may contain similar polyps, but also have finer, softer papillae, the consistency of which reflects neoplastic cell proliferation. Polyps and papillae of the same types are found on the surface of the ovary when the tumours are growing exophytically. True (invasive) serous carcinomas may be predominantly cystic or predominantly solid and may or may not contain grossly visible papillae.

On microscopical examination, the benign serous tumours are characterised by a single or pseudostratified layer of cells which typically bear cilia but may have an indifferent appearance. In borderline tumours, there is cellular proliferation and atypicality without 'destructive' invasion of the stromal component of the tumour (Fig. 2.1). The term 'destructive' invasion is confusing because borderline tumours may show a regular intrusion of small glandular structures with papillae into the stroma without recognisably altering it. This pseudoinvasion is in contrast to the disorderly true invasion of a serous carcinoma, which is often accompanied by a desmoplastic stromal reaction (Fig. 2.2). Serous borderline tumours often retain, at least focally, the cellular ciliation that is encountered in their benign counterparts, but most of their cells lack this feature. Also, these tumours often contain cells which secrete abundant mucin. In contrast to tumours in the mucinous category, however, the mucin in serous tumours is typically secreted from the surfaces of the cells, with very little accumulation within the upper part of their cytoplasm. Serous carcinomas lose even more of the endosalpingeal characteristics of benign serous tumours. The principal diagnostic features of these carcinomas are fine papillarity, irregular, often slit-like glandular lumens and psammoma bodies. The latter, though characteristic, are not specific for serous carcinomas, as they may be seen in a wide variety of other ovarian neoplasms, both benign and malignant and in inflammatory and other non-neoplastic conditions involving the surface epithelium. Serous adenofibromas or cystadenofibromas are usually benign, but may also be borderline or malignant. Although data are not available from a large series

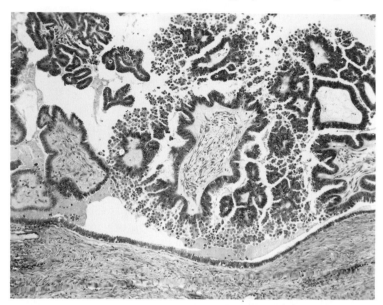

Fig. 2.1 Serous papillary cystadenoma of borderline malignancy (× 80). Characteristic cellular buds appear to float free in the lumen; there is no invasion of the cyst wall. Reproduced with permission from Serov et al 1973

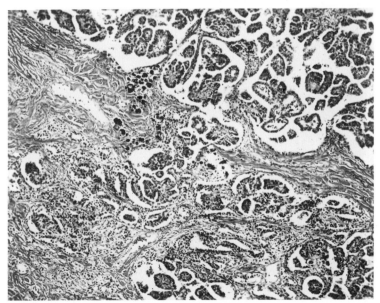

Fig. 2.2 Serous papillary adenocarcinoma (× 95). Clusters of tumour cells irregularly infiltrate the dense stroma. Reproduced with permission from Scully 1970

of cases, the impression exists that the presence of a predominant stromal component may interfere with the ability of the tumour cells to spread beyond the ovary.

Mucinous tumours

Benign and borderline mucinous tumours are almost always cystic and are typically multilocular. Mucinous carcinomas may be predominantly cystic or predominantly solid. In contrast to serous tumours, which tend to be relatively uniform throughout, mucinous tumours more often contain benign, borderline and malignant components within a single specimen. This finding emphasises the importance of meticulous gross examination and judicious sampling of these tumours to ensure an accurate diagnosis. The epithelial lining of mucinous cystadenomas, or the much rarer adenofibromas, usually resembles endocervical epithelium, but may have the appearance of intestinal epithelium with goblet cells, occasionally argentaffin cells, and rarely Paneth cells. The borderline and invasive forms of mucinous tumours are much more likely to contain intestinal type epithelium.

The distinction between mucinous cystadenomas of borderline malignancy and mucinous cystadenocarcinomas is more complicated and less sharp than in cases of serous tumours of analagous types. Whereas serous borderline tumours typically grow in the form of large cysts, sometimes with regular downgrowth of glands containing papillae into the underlying stroma, mucinous tumours, both borderline and invasive, may be characterised by large numbers of locules and glands, lying in stroma which resemble ovarian stroma. When these structures are lined by atypical cells and are not associated with a desmoplastic stromal response, it may be difficult to determine whether they are truly invasive or reflect only budding or benign intrusion into the stroma.

In view of this difficulty, Hart & Norris (1972) devised an elaborate set of criteria for distinguishing borderline from invasive mucinous tumours. Their criteria were as follows: if there is obvious invasion of the stroma, the tumour is a carcinoma; if there is no, or only equivocal evidence of invasion, the diagnosis rests on the height of the atypical cells lining the glands; and if the atypical nuclei are three or less in stratification, the tumour is considered borderline (Fig. 2.3), if four or greater, carcinoma (Fig. 2.4). Hart (1977) later added the finding of a cribriform pat-

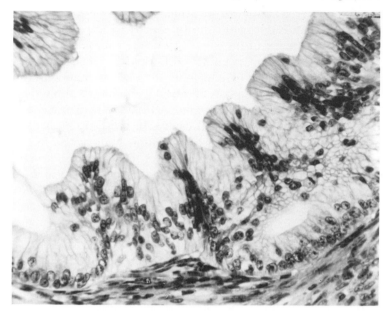

Fig. 2.3 Mucinous cystadenoma of borderline malignancy (× 350). Atypical nuclei are under four in height; stromal invasion is absent. Reproduced with permission from Serov et al 1973

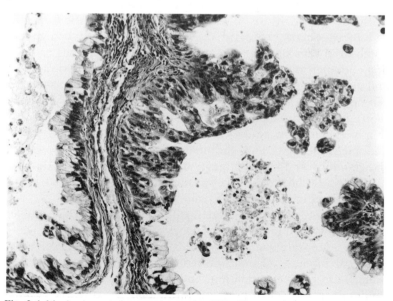

Fig. 2.4 Mucinous cystadenocarcinoma (× 120). Very atypical nuclei form thick layer lining cyst; pale intracellular mucin is visible in cells lining cyst on left. Reproduced with permission from Serov et al 1973

tern as another criterion for invasion. Although the approach of these investigators does not conform strictly to the concept of the presence or absence of invasion as the sole diagnostic criterion, the results of follow-up examination in their series justify its use.

A rare complication of mucinous tumours is pseudomyxoma peritonei, in which large pools of mucin, containing scattered neoplastic cells, lie in cysts and pockets surrounded by dense connective tissue within the peritoneal cavity. In most instances of this disorder, the ovarian tumour is of borderline malignancy. In many cases, the patient also has a mucocele of the appendix, which on microscopical examination, has an appearance identical to the ovarian tumour. In such cases, it appears most likely that the latter reflects metastasis from the former, but there is no consensus on the relation of the two lesions.

Endometrioid tumours

Endometrioid tumours are characterised by tubular glands, lined by stratified non-mucin-containing epithelium in well-differentiated areas. These tubular glands have the characteristic appearance of those within a proliferative endometrium. Unless one considers endometriosis, including its pseudoneoplastic form, the endometriotic or chocolate cyst, truly neoplastic, benign endometrioid tumours are very rare. They include lesions resembling endometrioid polyps, which may arise in endometriotic cysts and endometrioid adenofibromas, some of which show squamous neometaplasia (adenocanthofibromas) (Mostoufizadeh & Scully 1980). Endometrioid tumours of borderline malignancy include the relatively rare low-grade carcinomas that are confined within endometriotic cysts and endometrioid adenofibromas in which the glandular epithelium appears malignant but does not destructively invade the stroma. These tumours are so rare that at the present time, very little can be said about their prognosis.

Endometrioid carcinoma is defined as a tumour which resembles one of the typical forms of carcinoma of the endometrium. These include adenocarcinomas of various grades (Fig. 2.5), secretory adenocarcinomas, adenoacanthomas and adenosquamous carcinomas. On gross examination, endometrioid carcinomas may be predominantly cystic or predominantly solid. Usually, they do not possess distinctive gross features, except for the rare examples that

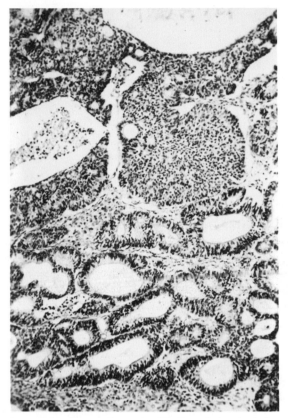

Fig. 2.5 Endometrioid adenocarcinoma (× 80). Rounded and tubular glands and solid masses of tumor cells are visible. Reproduced with permission from Scully 1968

arise from the linings of endometriotic cysts. In such cases, a typical chocolate cyst contains a papillary, or cauliflower-like, growth within its lumen, accompanied by varying degrees of invasion of the underlying wall. Up to one-third of endometrioid carcinomas of the ovary are accompanied by carcinomas of the uterine corpus, which typically resemble the ovarian tumours on microscopical examination. There is strong evidence to suggest that when this combination exists, it reflects independent primary growth in both organs, except in occasional cases where there is advanced growth in one organ and obvious spread to the other. The evidence for this conclusion is the only slightly less favourable prognosis when both organs are involved, compared to when the tumour is con-

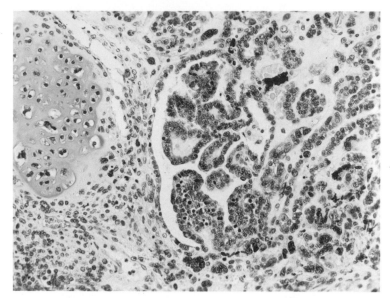

Fig. 2.6 Malignant mesodermal mixed tumour (× 160). Island of atypical cartilage lies on left; papillary adenocarcinoma is visible at centre. Reproduced with permission from Serov et al 1973

fined to the ovary. Therefore, in most cases of combined neoplasia, it would be more accurate to speak of a FIGO stage I ovarian carcinoma, plus a stage I corpus carcinoma, rather than a FIGO stage IIA ovarian carcinoma or a stage III corpus carcinoma.

Mixed epithelial and stromal tumours of endometrioid type, or pure endometrial stromal tumours of the ovary, are also included in the endometrioid category. Highly malignant (homogous) carcinosarcomas and malignant (heterologous) mesodermal mixed tumours (Fig. 2.6) are occasionally encountered, and mesodermal adenosarcomas and endometrioid stromal sarcomas, of varying degrees of malignancy, are less common. Malignant mesodermal mixed tumours must be differentiated from immature teratomas. The former occur almost exclusively in postmenopausal and menopausal women, and contain tissue elements which are entirely derivable from the mesoderm. In contrast, immature teratomas are encountered almost entirely in females under the age of 50 years, and contain elements derived from all three germ cell layers, with conspicuous ectodermal, particularly neuroectodermal, components.

Clear cell tumours

Clear cell tumours are characterised mainly by the presence of clear cells and/or hobnail cells (Figs 2.7, 2.8). The latter have bulbous nuclei that protrude into the lumens of tubules and cysts beyond the apparent cytoplasmic limits of the cells. The clear cells

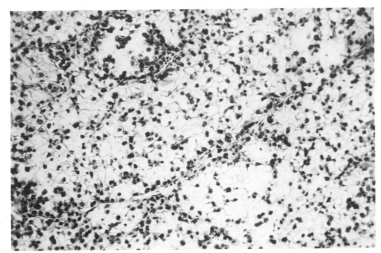

Fig. 2.7 Clear cell carcinoma (× 100). Clear polyhedral cells are arranged in a diffuse pattern. Reproduced with permission from Scully 1968

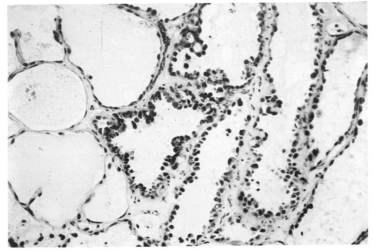

Fig. 2.8 Clear cell adenocarcinoma (× 170). Tubules and cysts are lined by hobnail cells. Reproduced with permission from Scully & Barlow 1967

may grow in solid masses or line glandular spaces. Occasionally, a highly papillary pattern is encountered. Rare tumours growing in the form of adenofibromas may be of benign or borderline malignancy, but most neoplasms in the clear cell category are carcinomas.

Except for their rare development within endometriotic cysts, clear cell carcinomas do not have distinctive gross features, sometimes being predominantly solid, and occasionally, mainly cystic. Although once considered mesonephric in origin and designated mesonephric or mesonephroid carcinoma, the clear cell carcinoma is now almost universally regarded as being of Mullerian nature, closely related to the endometrioid carcinoma. Clear cell carcinoma is associated with ovarian and pelvic endometriosis more frequently than any other tumour type, including the endometrioid carcinomas, with which it is occasionally admixed. Clear cell carcinomas also arise in the endometrium where, again, they may be admixed with typical forms of endometrial carcinoma. Finally, these tumours are encountered occasionally in the vaginas of young females who have been exposed prenatally to diethylstilboestrol and have a Mullerian type of adenosis, from which the neoplasms appear to originate (Scully 1981a). Although the cells of the clear cell carcinoma are generally considered to be Mullerian, their exact counterparts in the normal female genital tract are unknown. The clear and the hobnail cells, however, do closely resemble similar cells which are found in the endometrium during pregnancy, with the latter type of cell being a characteristic finding of the Arias-Stella phenomenon.

Brenner tumours

The Brenner tumour is a relatively frequent form of common epithelial tumour, but is usually encountered as an incidental finding at operation or in the pathology laboratory and not as a clinically detectable mass. The majority of these tumours are benign, appearing grossly as solid, white or pale yellow, discrete fibroma-like masses. On microscopical examination, islands of transitional epithelium lie within an abundant stroma which resemble fibromas, or occasionally, thecomas. In about one-third of the cases, mucinous glands or cysts are found within the transitional cell islands or separately in the stroma.

Brenner tumours of borderline malignancy, sometimes referred to as proliferative Brenner tumours, are typically multicystic with papillomatous growths within cysts. Microscopical examination reveals, in addition to benign Brenner neoplasia, intracystic papillary growth which closely resembles non-invasive grade I papillary transitional cell carcinoma of the urinary bladder. Some authors have criticised the use of the term borderline for these tumours on the grounds that none of them has been proven clinically malignant. Nevertheless, the follow-up has been short in many cases described in the literature, and one tumour reported as proliferating was later found to be complicated by liver metastases.

Malignant Brenner tumours are characterised by the presence of invasive transitional or squamous cell carcinoma, sometimes containing mucinous elements, in addition to benign Brenner neoplasia. Presence of the latter is a sine qua non for the diagnosis, since a number of poorly differentiated and undifferentiated carcinomas of the ovary have some resemblance to transitional or squamous cell carcinoma. Most tumours with such an appearance are poorly differentiated serous or endometrioid carcinomas. Malignant Brenner tumours may be predominantly solid or predominantly cystic, having no distinctive gross features.

Undifferentiated carcinoma

The term undifferentiated carcinoma has been applied by the WHO to carcinomas with minimal or no differentiation. The presence of occasional non-specific structures such as psammoma bodies, glands, or droplets or pools of mucin does not warrant placing the tumour in a more specific category. Most undifferentiated carcinomas are probably undifferentiated forms of serous or endometrioid carcinoma, since areas with similar patterns are commonly encountered in grade IV tumours of those types. However, within the undifferentiated category, bizarre-appearing neoplasms of an uncertain origin also exist. One subtype which has been recently segregated from others in the group is a small cell undifferentiated form which is encountered in older children and young women in the reproductive age group (Dickersin et al 1981). This tumour is notable for its frequent association with hypercalcemia, which disappears after removal of the tumour. Undifferentiated carcinomas are non-specific in their gross appearance, showing varying combinations of solid and cystic growth.

Mixed epithelial tumours

The diagnosis of a mixed epithelial tumour is warranted only when there is a quantitatively significant component of a second or third cell type within a common epithelial tumour. Notable, but rare examples of mixed epithelial tumours are mucinous cystadenoma and endometriosis, serous adenofibroma and endometriosis, and endometrioid and clear cell adenocarcinoma. Although the Brenner tumour often contains mucinous and, occasionally, serous elements, the presence of these components is by custom not considered sufficient to classify the tumour in the mixed category.

Sex cord-stromal tumours

Although the origins of the various cellular elements that make up the hormone-secreting compartment of the ovarian parenchyma are still in dispute, it is generally accepted that groups of cells in the developing gonads that have been called sex cords give rise to the granulosa cells of the ovary and the Sertoli cells of the testis. Likewise, the gonadal mesenchyme, or stroma, is the source of the ovarian stromal cells and their thecal and luteal derivatives, as well as the Leydig cells of the testis. The sex cord-stromal tumour category includes all neoplasms which contain these various cellular elements alone, or in combination, and in varying degrees of differentation. Many of these tumours produce steroid hormones but the most common form, the fibroma, is without endocrine function. As a group, sex cord-stromal tumours account for approximately 6% of ovarian neoplasms, and less than 10% of ovarian cancers.

Granulosa cell tumours

Granulosa cell tumours account for about 2% of all ovarian neoplasms and less than 10% of all ovarian cancers. The majority of these tumours are associated with oestrogenic effects, manifested in decreasing order of frequency, by postmenopausal bleeding, irregular bleeding or amenorrhoea during the reproductive era, and sexual pseudoprecocity. The most commonly associated pathological change is cystic hyperplasia of the endometrium, often with varying degrees of precancerous atypicality. About 4% of granulosa cell tumours are accompanied by carcinoma of the endometrium, which is typically low grade.

Ten to 15% of granulosa cell tumours are too small to be felt on pelvic examination but the remainder attain a larger size and are palpable, sometime even on abdominal examination. These tumours vary widely in their gross appearance. They may form solid masses composed of gray, white or yellow, firm or soft tissue, multilocular cysts with compartments filled with fluid or clotted blood, or unilocular cysts resembling serous cystadenomas. In other words, they may simulate grossly almost any type of ovarian neoplasm. On microscopical examination, most granulosa cell tumours contain varying numbers of fibroblasts or theca cells of ovarian stromal origin. The granulosa cells may form microfollicles (Call-Exner bodies, Fig. 2.9) or large follicles resembling cystic graafian follicles. The cells may also be arranged in diffuse masses, trabeculae, islands or cords. In addition to their characteristic patterns of growth, granulosa cells are usually recognisable by the appearance of their nuclei, which are typically round, oval or angular, pale and grooved. Juvenile granulosa cell tumours, which occur mostly in the first two decades, are characterised by greater immaturity of their cells, the formation of medium-sized

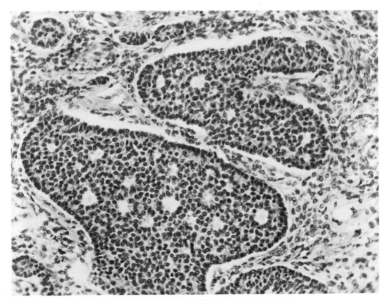

Fig. 2.9 Granulosa cell tumour (× 200). A microfollicular pattern with Call-Exner bodies is present. Reproduced with permission from Serov et al 1973

follicles containing mucin, and often extensive luteinisation of both their granulosal and thecal components. All granulosa cell tumours are considered potentially malignant. It is difficult to predict the prognosis in individual cases, but in general, neoplasms that are of a high histological grade and show considerable mitotic activity are more likely to recur, sometimes many years after surgery.

Tumours in thecoma-fibroma group

These tumours are so classified because both the typical fibroma and the typical thecoma are derivatives of the ovarian stromal cell, and an intermediate zone exists between them in which precise classification is impossible. Characteristically, fibromas are solid neoplasms composed of chalky-white, hard fibrous tissue, whereas thecomas are more likely to be softer and uniformly yellow, or white and flecked with yellow areas. Either tumour may contain areas of oedema or cystic degeneration. On microscopical examination, the fibroma resembles fibromas elsewhere in the body, typically containing intersecting fascicles of spindle-shaped fibroblasts that produce collagen (Fig. 2.10), and occasionally, a sto-

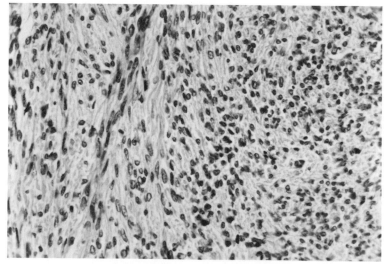

Fig. 2.10 Fibroma (× 325). The tumour is composed of intersecting fascicles of fibroblasts, which have produced collagen. Reproduced with permission from Serov et al 1973

riform pattern is observed. Forty per cent of fibromas over 10 cm in diameter are accompanied by ascites, which are believed to be due to seepage of fluid from areas of oedema within the tumour (Samanth & Black 1970). Less than 1% of fibromas, in general, are associated with the Meigs syndrome (ascites and hydrothorax, usually right-sided, disappearing after removal of the tumour).

Thecomas contain fibroblast-type cells and rounded cells which contain lipid and resemble, to varying degrees, the theca interna cells of the graafian follicle (Fig. 2.11). When some of the cells have the appearance of the theca lutein cells of the corpus luteum, the designation luteinised thecoma is used. Typically, fibromas contain little or no intracytoplasmic lipid, whereas thecomas contain moderate to large amounts. Thecomas are associated with the same clinical syndromes that accompany the granulosa cell tumour, except for sexual pseudoprecocity. The morphological changes in the endometrium are likewise similar to those seen in cases of granulosa cell tumour.

Fibromas and thecomas are rarely malignant. On microscopical examination, fibrosarcomas of the ovary resemble cellular fibromas, but tend to have more pleomorphic nuclei, and typically con-

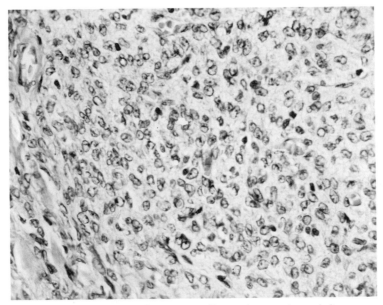

Fig. 2.11 Thecoma (× 380). The tumour cells are plump and rounded. Reproduced with permission from Scully 1979b

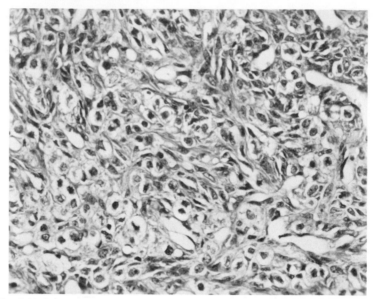

Fig. 2.12 Sclerosing stromal tumour (× 350). A disorderly mixture of spindle cells and rounded clear cells is present. Reproduced with permission from Chalvardjian & Scully 1973

tain four or more mitotic figures per 10 high-power fields (Prat & Scully 1981).

The tumours which have features between those of the fibroma and those of the thecoma are sometimes referred to as fibrothecomas or thecafibromas. One tumour in this category that has a distinctive microscopical appearance and age distribution is the sclerosing stromal tumour. It is characterised by an intimate, disorderly admixture of fibroblasts and theca cells (Fig. 2.12), often associated with cellular pseudolobules, which typically have a rich supply of thin-walled vessels. Dense sclerosis is a characteristic feature. Over 80% of the cases are found in the second and third decades, whereas less than 10% of fibromas and thecomas of the usual types are encountered in that age group. Grossly, the sclerosing stromal tumour forms a discrete whitish mass which is characteristically flecked with yellow and often shows areas of oedema and cyst formation. All reported examples have been benign.

Sertoli-Leydig cell tumours

Sertoli-Leydig cell tumours are much less common than those in the granulosa-stromal cell category, accounting for less than 1% of all ovarian neoplasms. These tumours show a wide variety of patterns and degrees of differentiation of their cellular components, and a small proportion of them also contain heterologous elements. The latter are most often glands and cysts lined by epithelium of gastrointestinal type, and less often masses of immature skeletal muscle or cartilage (Young et al 1982a, Prat et al 1982a).

On gross examination, Sertoli-Leydig cell tumours mimic granulosa cell tumours and thecomas in their various presentations. Microscopical examination reveals that Sertoli and Leydig cells exhibit varying degrees of maturity (Figs 2.13, 2.14). Sertoli cells may grow in the form of diffuse masses, trabeculae, islands, cords resembling sex cords, solid tubules, and/or hollow tubules. Leydig cells range from undifferentiated mesenchymal cells to mature-appearing cells in clusters, and rarely contain their specific intracytoplasmic inclusions, crystalloids of Reinke. All Sertoli Leydig cell tumours are considered potentially malignant. The poorly dif-

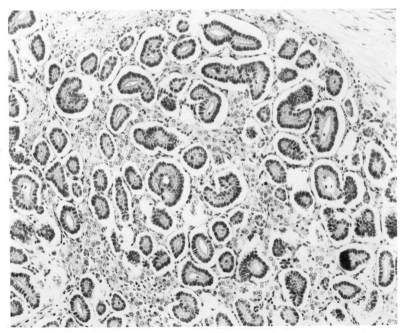

Fig. 2.13 Sertoli-Leydig cell tumour, well differentiated (× 130). Tubules are separated by masses of Leydig cells. Reproduced with permission from Morris & Scully 1958

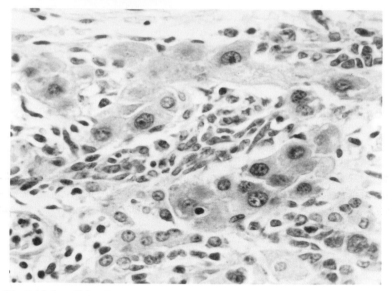

Fig. 2.14 Sertoli-Leydig cell tumour of intermediate differentiation (× 500). Small groups of immature Sertoli cells are separated by clusters of large Leydig cells. Reprouced with permission from Serov et al 1973

ferentiated forms, especially those with heterologous sarcomatous elements, have a poor prognosis. The outlook for patients with well-differentiated tumours is excellent. The majority of Sertoli-Leydig cell tumours are associated with virilisation due to the production of a variety of androgens by the Leydig cell component of the neoplasm. Some cases are, in contrast, non-functioning or associated with oestrogenic manifestations. The latter may result from oestrogen production by either the Sertoli or Leydig cell component, or from peripheral conversion to oestrone of the androgen, androstenedione, produced by the Leydig cell element.

Gynandroblastoma

This designation has been applied to tumours which contain cells of both testicular and ovarian types. Because of the great resemblance of granulosa and Sertoli cells, as well as theca and Leydig cells, there may be considerable subjectivity on the part of the pathologist in identifying them, whenever their distinctive features are lacking. Rarely do neoplasms fulfill the WHO criteria for the diagnosis of gynandroblastoma by possessing fully developed,

easily recognisable male and female cells, both in significant pro-
portions. Therefore, the existence of this tumour is mostly of
theoretical interest.

Sex cord-stromal tumours, unclassified

About 10% of ovarian neoplasms in the sex cord-stromal category
have cell types or patterns that are too poorly differentiated to
characterise specifically, or are between those of granulosa-
stromal and Sertoli-Leydig cell tumours. These neoplasms are
referred to as sex cord-stromal tumours, unclassified. Within this
category is a microscopically distinctive neoplasm designated sex
cord tumour with annular tubules (Young et al 1982b). It is characterised by simple and complex ring-shaped solid tubules which
have a pattern between that of a microfollicular granulosa cell
tumour and a solid-tubular Sertoli cell tumour (Figs 2.15, 2.16).
Areas of differentiation toward granulosa cell and Sertoli cell
neoplasia are often observed. Occasionally, this tumour is clinically malignant. It is usually non-functioning, but may be asso-

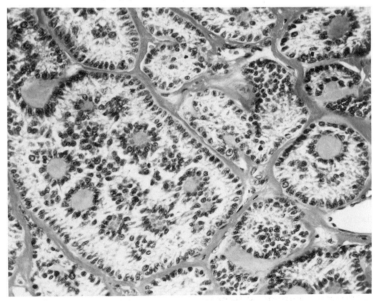

Fig. 2.15 Sex cord tumour with annular tubules (× 260). Simple and complex
tubules are present. The patient did not have the Peutz-Jeghers syndrome.
Reproduced with permission from Scully 1977b

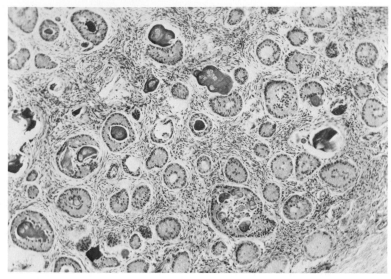

Fig. 2.16 Sex cord tumour with annular tubules (× 100). Calcification is prominent within the tubules, a characteristic of the cases associated with the Peutz-Jeghers syndrome. Reproduced with permission from Scully 1979b

ciated with oestrogenic manifestations. It is of considerable interest because when present in the form of multiple tumourlets in both ovaries, it is almost always associated with the Peutz-Jeghers syndrome. Likewise, it is almost always found on microscopical examination of the ovaries of patients with that disorder.

Lipid cell tumours

The terms lipid cell tumour and lipoid cell tumour have been used most often for ovarian neoplasms composed entirely of cells resembling typical steroid-hormone-producing cells, such as lutein cells, Leydig cells and adrenal cortical cells (Fig. 2.17). Since these tumours may contain little or no lipid, such designations are not always appropriate, and a term such as steroid cell tumour would be more desirable. When a neoplasm in this category is lipid-rich, it has an orange or yellow hue, but when it contains minimal quantities of lipid, or none at all, it tends to be reddish-brown, brown, or even black if the neoplastic cells contain large quantities of lipochrome pigment. Whenever a pathologist encounters a tumour in this grouping, all the clinical, biochemical, topographical, histological, and histochemical features should be examined to

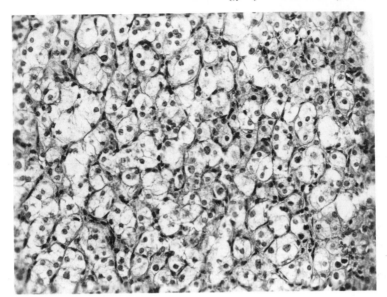

Fig. 2.17 Lipid cell tumour (× 100). The tumour cells are large and rounded and contain vacuolated cytoplasm. Reproduced with permission from Morris & Scully 1958

attempt to arrive at a more specific diagnosis, such as adrenal cortical rest tumour, Leydig cell tumour, which is usually of hilus cell origin, or stromal luteoma, a neoplasm of lutein cells.

Adrenal cortical rests, which have the appearance of a miniature encapsulated adrenal cortex on microscopical examination, have been identified in the broad ligament in 27% of hysterectomy specimens. Occasionally, these structures lie in the hilar region, and in extremely rare cases, in the stroma of the ovary. Although lipid cell tumours were at one time commonly designated as adrenal rest tumours, there is no well established case of an adrenal rest tumour of the ovary in the literature. The associated endocrine manifestations and hormone profiles, which have been used as evidence for an adrenal cortical origin of several examples of lipid cell tumour, are non-specific. There are, however, two unpublished cases in which cortisol production by such a tumour, associated with Cushing's syndrome was demonstrated. Whether this finding is absolute evidence of the adrenal cortical nature of a neoplasm remains debatable. From the topographical viewpoint, lipid cell tumours typically replace the ovary and are not in the broad ligament or hilus, strongly suggesting that their origin is not in adrenal cortical rests.

Hilus cells, or hilar Leydig cells, can be found in 80 to 85% of adult ovaries on careful sectioning, and, like the Leydig cells of the testis, can give rise to neoplasms. To diagnose a hilus cell tumour, the centring of the tumour in the hilus, and the presence of the specific crystalloids of Reinke in the cytoplasm of some of the cells must be established. If this is not done, the neoplasm cannot be distinguished with certainty from other tumours in the steroid cell category. An absence of crystalloids of Reinke does not exclude the hilus cell origin of a tumour, however, since these structures are said to be absent in 60% of Leydig cell tumours of the testis. Leydig cell tumours rarely arise directly from the ovarian stroma.

The ovarian stroma gives rise to the theca cells of the graafian follicle, which become luteinised in the corpus luteum, as well as to lutein cells in the stroma apart from the follicles. The latter cells are called luteinised stromal cells or stromal lutein cells, and their presence in more than minimal quantities is referred to as stromal hyperthecosis. Since most lipid cell tumours are centred in the ovary, it appears probable that they arise from neoplastic transformation of lutein cells, but it is only when the tumour is small and surrounded by ovarian stroma, and especially when stromal hyperthecosis is seen elsewhere, that one can be certain of the stromal origin of the tumour and the corresponding diagnosis of stromal luteoma.

In pregnancy, hyperplastic nodules of lutein cells, designated pregnancy luteomas, have been encountered, on rare occasions, during a caesarean section or tubal ligation. These nodules are not true neoplasms, but reflect a reversible proliferation of lutein cells that appears to depend on the high level of chorionic gonadotrophin which prevails during pregnancy. On microscopical examination, pregnancy luteomas may be difficult to distinguish from steroid cell tumours, but their multicentricity in at least one-third of the cases, their minimal content of lipid, and their frequent mitotic figures are helpful in the differential diagnosis. After pregnancy, these lesions typically undergo degenerative changes with lipid accumulation and fibrosis.

If a tumour or nodule of steroid-type cells cannot be proven to be in any of the above specific categories, it is placed in the unclassified or lipid cell group. Tumours of steroid cell type are usually virilising, but may be oestrogenic or non-functioning. In a series reported from the Armed Forces Institute of Pathology (Taylor & Norris 1967), approximately 25% were associated with a malignant behaviour. The malignant tumours were all 8 cm or greater, in diameter, and usually had malignant features cytologically, although the prognosis of these tumours is difficult to assess on microscopical examination alone. Leydig cell tumours which contain crystalloids of Reinke rarely have malignant behaviour.

Germ-cell tumours

Germ-cell tumours are among the most diverse and interesting of all ovarian neoplasms (Kurman & Norris 1977). They account for approximately 25% of the latter, largely due to the frequency of their most common subtype, the dermoid cyst, or mature cystic teratoma. Malignant forms of these tumours account for less than 3% of all ovarian cancers in the Western World. Germ-cell tumours are most often encountered in children and premenopausal women. Those that are discovered in older patients probably began to develop before the menopause, at a time when their cells of origin were still present within the ovary.

Dysgerminoma

Dysgerminoma, which accounts for approximately 50% of the malignant primitive germ-cell tumours of the ovary, is a uniform-appearing tumour made up of large, rounded polyhedral cells with abundant clear cytoplasm, and central nuclei containing one or a few prominent nucleoli (Fig. 2.18). The cytoplasmic clarity is due to a large content of glycogen. Various amounts of lymphocytes are usually present in the stroma of the tumour, and are also typically sprinkled among the neoplastic cells. Occasionally, non-caseating granulomas appear in the stroma. Varying numbers of mitotic figures are present, but their quantity has not been clearly related to the behaviour of the tumour. A rare subtype of dysgerminoma contains scattered multinucleated giant cells having the morphological features of syncytiotrophoblast cells. The presence of such cells is important because they may secrete chorionic gonadotrophin and result in oestrogenic or androgenic clinical manifestations. On gross examination, the dysgerminoma typically forms a large lobulated mass composed of pale yellow or cream-coloured tissue, which is soft or firm, depending on its content of fibrous stroma.

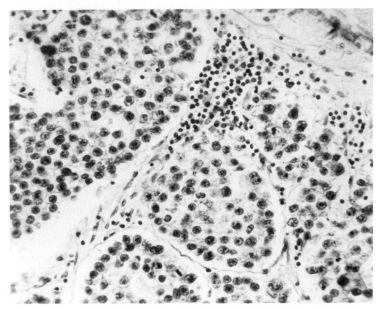

Fig. 2.18 Dysgerminoma (× 300). The nuclei are uniform and rounded. Stromal lymphocytes are visible in the upper part of the picture. Reproduced with permission from Scully 1963

Endodermal sinus tumour (yolk sac tumour)

This tumour, which was initially classified as a mesonephroma, accounts for approximately 20% of the primitive germ-cell tumours of the ovary. Careful investigation by the late Danish pathologist, Teilum (1965) demonstrated that its architecture simulates that of the labyrinthine placenta of the rodent, in which yolk sac diverticula (endodermal sinuses) invade the extraembryonic mesenchyme in the form of papillary projections with central capillaries (Schiller-Duval bodies, Fig. 2.19). Confirmation of the yolk sac nature of the tumour is afforded by its content of hyaline bodies that stain for alpha-1-antitrypsin, the demonstration of alpha-fetoprotein in its tumour cells, and the occasional growth pattern of polyvesicular vitelline tumour. In the latter, vesicles with eccentric constrictions recapitulate the division of the primary yolk sac vesicle of the embryo into a vestigial vesicle and a secondary definitive vesicle. The former undergoes atrophy, while the latter becomes the primitive gut of the embryo. Thus, it is not surprising that the endodermal sinus tumour contains not only elements

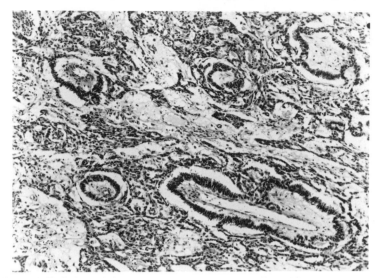

Fig ? 19 Endodermal sinus tumour (× 80). Single papillae with central vessels (Schiller-Duval bodies) protrude into spaces. Reproduced with permission from Serov et al 1973

resembling extraembryonic structures, but also embryonic components, usually in the form of glands lined by intestinal-type epithelium with goblet cells. Recently, a hepatoid form of yolk sac tumour has also been described, in which embryonic differentiation proceeds in the direction of the liver (Prat et al 1982b). Endodermal sinus tumours have a gross appearance that suggests a high degree of malignancy, being composed of gray to yellow tissue with areas of haemorrhage, necrosis, gelatinous degeneration and cyst formation. Rupture of the capsule is found in more than 25% of the cases at initial surgery (Kurman & Norris 1976a).

Embryonal carcinoma

The term embryonal carcinoma was once used as a synonym for endodermal sinus tumour, but subsequently, the two tumours have been shown to be distinct in both their morphological and clinical features (Kurman & Norris 1976b). The embryonal carcinoma accounts for only about 3% of the primitive germ-cell tumours of the ovary. On microscopical examination, it closely resembles the embryonal carcinoma which is encountered more frequently in the testis, being composed of solid masses, glandular arrangements and papillary formations composed of anaplastic cells, resembling those of the germ disc of the embryo. Isolated syncytiotrophoblast cells are found in almost all cases. The tumour is somewhat more frequent in children than the endodermal sinus tumour, and because of its secretion of chorionic gonadotrophin, it is capable of endocrine manifestations, most often sexual precocity in the child, but also menstrual disturbances, and rarely, androgenic changes in the adult. Typically, the chorionic gonadotrophin level in blood is elevated. The alpha-fetoprotein level may also be high, suggesting that some embryonal carcinomas contain morphologically unrecognisable endodermal elements.

Choriocarcinoma

Choriocarcinoma is composed of cytotrophoblasts and syncytiotrophoblasts, and is rarely encountered in its pure form. More often, it forms a small component of an embryonal carcinoma or teratoma. Since it secretes chorionic gonadotrophin, it may result in sexual pseudoprecocity in children, and menstrual abnormalities and androgenic changes in adults.

Polyembryoma

Polyembryoma is a very rare form of primitive germ-cell tumour which is characterised by a preponderant content of embryoid bodies resembling, to varying degrees, normal, early embryos. Foci of differentiation into teratomatous elements are seen in most cases. Because these tumours often contain trophoblastic elements, they may be associated with high levels of chorionic gonadotrophin and related endocrine manifestations.

Teratomas

At one time. teratomas were divided into two major categories: cystic and solid. The former were usually considered benign, and the latter almost always malignant. More recent investigation has shown that the behaviour of these tumours is more dependent on their microscopical than their gross characteristics. The modern classification of teratomas includes three major categories. Immature teratoma is defined as a tumour containing elements from all three embryonic layers, endoderm, mesoderm and ectoderm and including at least some immature elements. In contrast, the mature teratoma is composed exclusively of well-differentiated fetal to adult-type tissues. The third category, monodermal or monophyletic teratoma, includes those tumours in which there is a predominance of a single tissue element, which is generally highly differentiated, such as thyroid (struma ovarii), carcinoid, or very rarely, other types of tissue.

The immature teratoma accounts for almost 20% of primitive germ-cell tumours of the ovary, and typically, forms a predominantly solid mass with a heterogenous appearance on the sectioned surface. The solid tissue may be soft, generally reflecting the presence of neural tissue, or hard due to the presence of cartilaginous or bony elements. The cysts may be filled with serous or mucinous fluid or sebaceous material, which sometimes contains hair. On microscopical examination, the tumour may have a wide variety of components, some of which are almost always mature. The most prominent immature element in most cases is neuroectodermal, consisting of masses of primitive cells, which often have area of necrosis, foci of glial differentiation and neuroepithelial rosettes of ependymal type (Fig. 2.20). Immature teratomas have been graded from 1 to 3, depending on the degree and amount of immature tissue. This grading system has prognostic and therapeutic significance.

Mature teratomas that are predominantly solid, sometimes referred to as teratomas, grade 0, are composed exclusively of well-differentiated tissue, without mitotic activity. On gross examination, they are similar to immature teratomas, but are likely to contain less soft tissue and to be free of necrosis. Despite reports to the contrary, the mature solid teratoma is almost always, if not always, clinically benign, provided that adequate sectioning of the specimen has excluded the presence of immature elements, and justifies the designation, mature. Both immature and mature solid teratomas may spread to the peritoneum in the form of mature implants, which are usually composed exclusively of glial tissue. The presence of such implants does not appear to influence the prognosis, since patients having them have lived asymptomatically for many years without therapy.

The most common form of mature teratoma is cystic, usually a dermoid cyst, which accounts for over 20% of all ovarian tumours. This tumour is so named because its lining is composed predom-

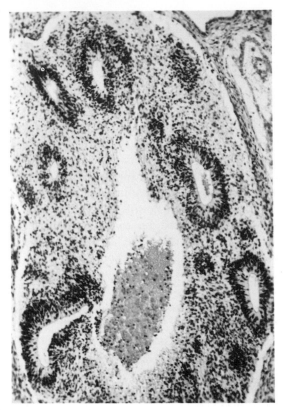

Fig. 2.20 Immature teratoma (× 110). Cellular glial tissue containing neuroepithelial rosettes is centrally necrotic. Reproduced with permission from Scully 1970

inantly of skin and its appendages, although portions may be lined by respiratory epithelium or glial tissue. However, the dermoid cyst is a true teratoma because it contains elements derived from mesoderm, endoderm and ectoderm in over two-thirds of the cases (Fig. 2.21). Generally, gross examination reveals a thin-walled cyst containing sebaceous material and hair. Typically, surgery discloses a localised solid protuberance known as the mammilla or Rokitanksy protuberance, which is generally composed mainly of adipose tissue. Bone and teeth may be observed in the wall of the cyst or protruding into its lumen. When a dermoid cyst ruptures, it can expel oily material into the surrounding tissue or into the peritoneal cavity, where it excites an inflammatory reaction with the eventual appearance of foreign-body giant cells and fibrosis. Secondary malignant change, generally of an adult-cancer

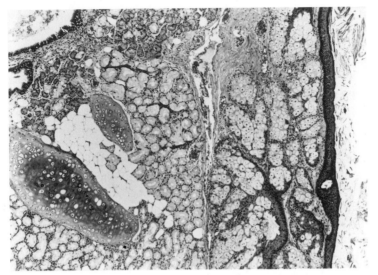

Fig. 2.21 Dermoid cyst (x 50). Two plates of cartilage border a pale island of fat; salivary gland tissue partly surrounds the cartilage and fat; glands are visible in the upper left portion of the picture. The cyst is lined by epidermis, under which numerous sebaceous glands lie. Reproduced with permission from Serov et al 1973

type, occurs in 1 to 2% of dermoid cysts. In about 80% of the cases, the malignant tumour is a squamous cell carcinoma, which appears as a fungating mass protruding into the lumen of the cyst, or an area of thickening in its wall. Much less often, the malignant change is a sarcoma of various types, an adenocarcinoma, a carcinoid, or other types of cutaneous malignancy, such as squamous cell carcinoma in situ, basal cell carcinoma or malignant melanoma.

A dermoid cyst rarely contains highly organised tissues such as a segment of colon, an appendix, or a malformed eye. The most highly developed form of mature teratoma resembles a human monster, and is referred to as a fetiform teratoma or homunculus.

Monodermal (monophyletic) teratomas

The most common monodermal teratoma is the struma ovarii. Although thyroid tissue can be identified on careful sectioning in up to 20% of dermoid cysts, the term struma is appropriate only when such tissue is grossly recognisable, or is the predominant or apparently sole component of a teratoma. On gross examination, thyroid tissue is easily recognisable as brown or greenish brown gelatinous tissue when it forms a mass adjacent to a dermoid cyst. More often than not, however, the tumour occurs in pure or almost pure form as a solid mass or a unilocular or multilocular cyst containing mucoid or gelatinous fluid. Grossly, the cystic struma is easily misinterpreted as a mucinous cystadenoma and is distinguishable from the latter mainly by its green to brown colour. On microscopical examination, the struma may resemble normal thyroid tissue or a thyroid adenoma, which may be macrofollicular, microfollicular, embryonal or mixed in type. On very rare occasions, a struma causes or contributes to the development of hyperthyroidism. Less than 5% of strumas are malignant in the form of either a follicular or a papillary carcinoma. Very few of these cases are well documented in the literature. A strumal adenoma may, in rare cases, implant on the peritoneum in the form of benign nodules of thyroid tissue, peritoneal strumosis, a condition that is compatible with longevity.

The second most common type of monodermal teratoma is the ovarian carcinoid, which is occasionally apparently pure, but is more often associated with grossly or microscopically demonstrable teratomatous elements. The primary ovarian carcinoid is usually of the insular or midgut type (Robboy et at 1975), but may be trabecular, with a ribbon-like pattern of growth (Robboy et al 1977). The insular carcinoid is accompanied by the carcinoid syndrome in approximately one-third of the cases. Unlike the vast majority of carcinoids, the ovarian form can produce the syndrome without metastasising, because its secretions are not routed through the portal venous system and detoxified by the liver. For that reason, it is associated with the only type of carcinoid syndrome that can be cured by removal of the primary tumour. The ovarian trabecular carcinoid has not been reported to be accompanied by the carcinoid syndrome. Although all carcinoids are potentially malignant, the ovarian type has an excellent prognosis with only rare examples resulting in metastases and eventual death. On microscopical examination, carcinoids have often been confused with granulosa cell and Sertoli cell tumours, but the architectural and cytological features of these tumours differ strikingly from those of carcinoids. The demonstration of argentaffin and/or argyrophil granules on special staining, or dense core granules on electron microscopical examination, provides confirmation of the diagnosis.

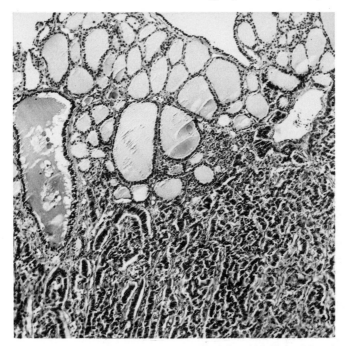

Fig. 2.22 Strumal carcinoid (× 100). Colloid-filled thyroid follicles (above) merge with trabecular carcinoid (below). Reproduced with permission from Morris & Scully 1958

A rare form of ovarian teratoma consists of struma and carcinoid, which may be associated as a combination tumour or a single mass of intimately admixed components (Robboy & Scully 1980). In this neoplasm, thyroid acini and carcinoid, which are typically of the trabecular variety, coexist (Fig. 2.22). The latter may invade the former in such a way that the colloid material becomes surrounded by argyrophil or argentaffin cells. The strumal carcinoid has not been associated with the carcinoid syndrome, but evidence of thyroid hyperfunction has been suggested in occasional cases. Like pure primary carcinoids of the ovary, this tumour has almost always been clinically benign.

Very rare forms of monodermal teratoma include neuroectodermal malignant tumours which resemble primitive malignant tumours of the central nervous system (Aguirre & Scully 1982), sebaceous gland neoplasms and retinal anlage tumours.

Mixed malignant germ-cell tumours

Mixed malignant germ-cell tumours account for about 8% of malignant primitive germ-cell tumours of the ovary (Kurman & Norris 1976c), and their occurrence emphasises the importance of careful gross examination of germ-cell tumours and judicious sampling of them for microscopical examination. Investigation has shown that the prognosis in cases of mixed germ-cell neoplasia depends not only on the nature of the malignant elements identified, but also on their quantity.

Tumours associated with abnormal sexual development

Several types of gonadal tumours have been associated occasionally, and a few types almost exclusively, with abnormal gonadal development. In many instances, these tumours have replaced the involved gonad so that its identity as an ovary, testis, or developmentally abnormal gonad has been impossible to determine. When such tumours develop in phenotypic females, they are conveniently classified among ovarian neoplasms. The following account will review the types of gonadal neoplasia which occur in the various forms of abnormal sexual development in the phenotypic female (Scully 1981b). Although testicular tumours of steroid cell type which behave physiologically like adrenal cortical tumours occur in the adrenogenital syndrome occasionally, particularly in the salt-losing form, only one similar ovarian tumour has been reported.

Patients with testicular feminisation, or the androgen insensitivity syndrome, are phenotypic females with a 46 XY karyotype and cryptorchids, containing tubules and Leydig cells which resemble those of the fetal testis and a stroma which is indistinguishable from ovarian stroma. Patients with this disorder have the appearance of females because their end organs fail to respond to androgens; but, because their testes produce normal or almost normal Mullerian-inhibiting substance, the fallopian tubes, uterus and the upper part of the vagina are absent. Despite the fact that they have testes, affected patients are most often seen by gynaecologists because of primary amenorrhoea or the development of an adnexal mass. Typically, the masses are Sertoli cell adenomas, which may attain diameters of over 20 cm, germinomas (seminomas), or rarely, other types of malignant germ-cell tumour. These tumours rarely develop before puberty. Seminomas are found in less than one-third of the patients with this syndrome by the age of 50 years. This frequency of late cancer development warrants orchidectomy once pubertal development has been achieved.

Other phenotypic females, most of whom are masculinised and have a Y chromosome, usually with a 46 XY, but occasionally with a 45X/46XY, or other mosaic karyotype, often show partial or complete replacement of one or both gonads by gonadoblastomas, or by common germ-cell tumours, usually germinomas. Patients with these karyotypes may have pure gonadal dysgenesis with bilateral streak gonads, mixed gonadal dysgenesis with a streak on one side and a testis, usually dysgenetic, on the other; or dysgenetic male pseudohermaphroditism with malformed testes on both sides. The gonadoblastoma, which is often of very small size, is composed of two and usually three of the constituents of the developing gonad, germ-cells, immature sex cord elements of Sertoli or granulosa type, and Leydig or lutein cells. The tumour exhibits several types of relation of the germ cells and immature sex cord elements, and is often calcified (Fig. 2.23). The gonadoblastoma is typically an in situ form of germ-cell malignancy, since

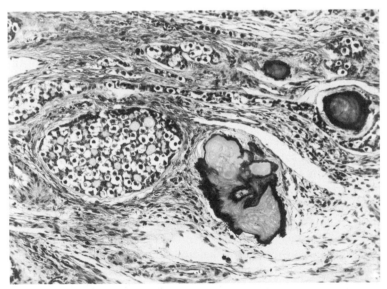

Fig. 2.23 Gonadoblastoma (× 130). Cellular nests composed of germ cells and smaller sex-cord cells and masses of calcification are present. Reproduced with permission from Serov et al 1973

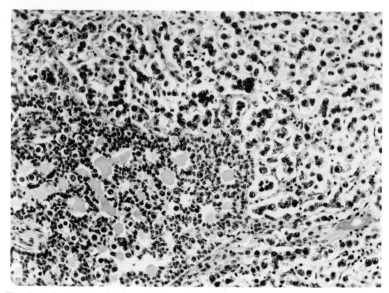

Fig. 2.24 Gonadoblastoma with dysgerminoma (× 160). Gonadoblastoma with hyaline bodies (left) lies adjacent to dysgerminoma on right. Reproduced with permission from Serov et al 1973

it has rarely been reported to metastasise. Half of the cases, however, are complicated by invasive germinoma (Fig. 2.24) and many fewer by other types of malignant germ-cell tumour development. Because of its content of Leydig of lutein cells, the gonadoblastoma may function, most often by producing androgens, but occasionally oestrogens, or both. Germinomas, as well as other types of malignant germ-cell tumours, may occasionally be encountered in pure form in phenotypic females with dysgenetic gonads, but it is possible in such cases that an underlying gonadoblastoma was destroyed by the tumour or overlooked because of inadequate sampling. Gonadoblastomas occur very rarely in patients with 45 X Turner's syndrome, in patients with a 46 XX karyotype, or in true hermaphrodites.

A mixed tumour consisting of sex cord elements and germ cells, rarely simulates a gonadoblastoma, but arises in the ovary of an otherwise normal female. Most of the reported cases of this tumour have been described by Talerman (1972). They tend to occur in infants and children but may develop in adults. Unlike the gonadoblastoma, they are not usually associated with calcification, and in some cases, show a wide variety of patterns and recapitulating testicular development.

Metastatic tumours

Almost every type of tumour has been reported to metastasise to
the ovary, but the great frequency of secondary ovarian involvement observed at autopsy does not reflect the frequency of ovarian
metastases which present clinically as ovarian cancer. The same
can be said for series of metastatic ovarian cancer cases encountered by the surgical pathologist, since a relatively high proportion
of these will be metastases of breast origin that have been discovered incidentally during a therapeutic oophorectomy. If one considers only those cases of metastatic tumour which present
clinically as adnexal masses, these account for about 8% of ovarian
cancers. The vast majority of these originate in the gastrointestinal
tract, more often in the large intestine than the stomach. Metastases of large-intestinal origin may be solid and composed of soft
and friable or firm and gritty tissue, but more often are multicystic.
Most of the cysts are the result of haemorrhage and necrosis, but
some are thin-walled and filled with mucus. Microscopical examination reveals a picture similar to that of primary adenocarcinomas of the large intestine. Glandular structures are typically lined
by poorly differentiated epithelium which is secreting mucin into
the lumens. Goblet cells are occasionally seen in the lining epithelium and necrosis is a common feature. Metastases from the
stomach, in contrast, are typically solid, rarely contain cysts, and
may also be thin-walled and filled with mucus. On microscopical
examination, most of these tumours are characterised, at least
partially, by the proliferation of signet cells and small acini lined
with mucin-rich epithelium scattered in a sarcomatoid stroma
(Fig. 2.25). This pattern was first described by Krukenberg, and
subsequently, his name was assigned to the tumour. In addition
to the features that he described, larger glands, which may have
a tubular configuration (Bullon et al 1981), cysts, and solid areas
of neoplastic cell growth may be observed. Occasionally, Krukenberg tumours originate from a large-intestinal carcinoma, a breast
carcinoma, or rarely, a neoplasm in another organ which is capable of giving rise to a mucin-producing tumour. Conversely, a
metastatic carcinoma from the stomach occasionally lacks the features of a Krukenberg tumour. Sectioning of a Krukenberg tumour reveals soft or firm, sometimes fibromatous tissue which is
typically the site of oedema, mucinous degeneration, necrosis or
a combination of these changes.
    Carcinomas of the female genital tract may spread directly to

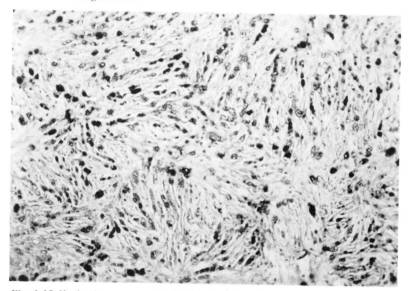

Fig. 2.25 Krukenberg tumour (× 100). The dark cells are signet-ring cells stained with periodic acid-Schiff method, lying in abundant pale stroma. Reproduced with permission from Scully 1979b

an ovary in their advanced stages. Involvement in cases of vulvar, vaginal and cervical carcinoma is rare. Ovarian carcinoma of the endometrioid type is encountered in approximately 10% of cases of carcinoma of the endometrium, but in the great majority of such cases, the evidence suggests that the ovarian tumour is an independent primary carcinoma rather than a metastatic deposit. Carcinomas of the fallopian tube may extend directly to the ipsilateral ovary. Occasionally, when the tube and ovary are converted into a single, solid or cystic neoplastic mass, it is impossible to determine which site is primary. In such cases, the term tubo-ovarian carcinoma has been used.

A few other very rare forms of ovarian metastatic disease deserve mention. Disseminated carcinoma of the breast is encountered in approximately 25% of therapeutic oophorectomy specimens, usually in the form of multiple, varisized firm to hard nodules. Rarely, breast carcinoma presents clinically as an ovarian mass without an apparent primary tumour (Young et al 1981). In some of these cases, the breast has not been examined adequately, whereas in others, only careful investigation has revealed the presence of a carcinoma. In unusual cases, a carcinoid tumour, most often from the ileum, presents clinically as an ovarian mass (Robboy et al 1974). The metastatic carcinoid can closely simulate a primary ovarian tumour because it typically elicits an extensive fibromatous response on the part of the ovarian stroma, creating a gross resemblance to a fibroma. Sometimes, cyst formation takes place and the tumour has an appearance similar to that of a cystadenofibroma. On microscopical examination, the carcinoid may consist of small islands or long ribbons of argentaffin or argyrophil cells separated by a stroma of varying amounts. In doubtful cases, staining for argentaffin and argyrophil granules facilitates the diagnosis. Often, a mass is evident in the ileum or its mesentery at the time of surgery, but a primary tumour in that location may be small and easily overlooked, or the source of the neoplasm may be another organ. Melanomas and renal cell carcinomas are among other tumours which, on extremely rare occasions, present as ovarian masses. The former must be distinguished from primary malignant melanomas of germ-cell origin, and the latter from clear cell carcinomas of the ovary.

Ovarian lymphomas are generally considered to be in the category of metastatic or secondary tumours, but on occasion, appear to be primary. They generally form large fleshy masses. A common form is the Burkitt lymphoma, which is encountered mainly in Africa. Lymphomas rarely present as ovarian masses in other parts of the world. Several types have been described, particularly the histiocytic and poorly differentiated lymphocytic. Ovarian lymphomas are often misdiagnosed as undifferentiated carcinoma, dysgerminoma, or granulosa cell tumour, particularly because their growth patterns in the dense ovarian stroma may differ from those observed in lymph nodes, i.e., the cells may be compartmentalised into discrete islands and rows instead of growing diffusely.

Ovarian tumours with functioning stroma

Almost all types of ovarian neoplasm, benign and malignant, primary and metastatic, have been reported on occasion to be associated with androgenic, oestrogenic, or progestagenic manifestations, based on stimulation of their stroma to differentiate into lutein cells. These 'ovarian tumours with functioning stroma' fall into three major categories — those in which trophoblastic cells within the tumour secrete chorionic gonadotrophin, which is present in high quantities locally and stimulates the stroma; those occurring during pregnancy when high levels of chorionic gonadotrophin in the blood stimulate the tumour stroma, and an idiopathic group. Tumours which contain trophoblastic elements include choriocarcinoma, embryonal carcinoma, polyembryoma and dysgerminoma with syncytiotrophoblast cells (Zaloudek et al 1981). These tumours have been associated with both oestrogenic and androgenic manifestations. A wide variety of tumours occurring during pregnancy have been accompanied by virilisation. Other tumours in this category are possibly oestrogenic, but have no clinical effect because of an already existing high oestrogen level. There is ample clinical, biochemical, histological and histochemical evidence that the function of tumours occurring during pregnancy depends on the circulating chorionic gonadotrophin.

Tumours with functioning stroma are most often in the idiopathic group. Although their androgenic or oestrogenic manifestations are occasionally overt, more often, their activity is evident only at a subclinical level. Investigation of steroid hormone metabolites in the urine of patients with common epithelial tumours suggests that up to 40% are associated with elevated total urinary oestrogens and/or pregnanediol (Rome et al 1981). The mechanism of the stromal stimulation in this idiopathic group of functioning tumours is unclear. It is interesting that certain types of tumour, such as primary and metastatic mucin-secreting neoplasms, are much more likely to result in stromal stimulation with hormone production than non-mucin-secreting neoplasms. Kurman (1975) has shown that some tumours in the idiopathic group contain neoplastic epithelial cells which stain positively for chorionic gonadotrophin by immunohistochemical methods. In other cases, however, the results have been negative. Although mechanical effects on the stroma have been postulated as the explanation for hormone production by the proliferating stromal cells, it appears more likely that an inductive substance of unknown type, in some cases chorionic gonadotrophin, is responsible for this phenomenon.

Tumour-like conditions

Various inflammatory and proliferative lesions of the ovary and adjacent areas can simulate ovarian tumours. Some of these require special mention because of their close resemblance to ovarian neoplasia, even after close surgical inspection. The frequently encountered solitary follicle cyst and corpus luteum cyst are typically thin-walled and rarely exceed 8 cm in diameter. The solitary luteinised follicle cysts of late pregnancy and the puerperium, however, may attain a giant size (Clement & Scully 1980).

Multiple follicle cysts can develop in otherwise normal ovaries, in ovaries affected by pelvic inflammatory disease or in the Stein-Leventhal syndrome. The last disorder is typically manifested by bilateral ovarian enlargement, whitish thickening of the outer cortices and multiple follicle cysts that form just below the surfaces in a clinical setting of anovulation and infertility. Rarely, ovarian tumours may occur in polycystic ovaries and distort their appearance.

Hyperreactio luteinalis, or the ovarian hyperstimulation syndrome, is most often a complication of trophoblastic disease of the uterus, but occasionally, it is seen in cases of fetal hydrops or in association with a normal pregnancy. Finally, it may result from the administration of ovulation inducing drugs. In hyperreactio luteinalis, both ovaries may be greatly enlarged by stromal oedema and multiple luteinised follicle cysts, which are often filled with blood. Another tumour-like condition associated with pregnancy is the pregnancy luteoma, which occurs almost exclusively during the third trimester and which is accompanied by virilisation in about 25% of the cases. This lesion depends on circulating chorionic gonadotrophin for both its structural and functional integrity. Typically, solid nodules, which may attain a diameter of 20 to 30 cm, are encountered. They are multiple in approximately one-third of the cases and bilateral in at least one-quarter. Microscopical examination discloses a proliferation of large steroid-type cells. After the completion of pregnancy, these cells undergo fatty degeneration and involute very much like degenerating corpora lutea.

Proliferative lesions of the ovarian stroma can also resemble tumours. These include the closely related disorders, hyperplasia, hyperthecosis and massive oedema. Ovarian stromal hyperplasia of varying degrees is a common phenomenon that reaches its peak in the early postmenopausal years. It may be focal and nodular, or diffusely enlarge both ovaries. Whether it has any endocrine significance has not been determined with certainty. The hyperplastic stroma may contain varying numbers of nests of lutein cells (luteinised stromal cells). When these are present in more than minimal numbers, the disorder is known as stromal hyperthecosis. It may occur in women of all ages and can be associated with androgenic and/or oestrogenic manifestations. When it develops in patients in the reproductive age group, it may produce the clinical picture of the Stein-Leventhal syndrome or masculinisation, which is often complicated by obesity, hypertension, impaired glucose tolerance, hyperplasia or even carcinoma of the endometrium. Stromal hyperplasia and hyperthecosis are almost always bilateral and may enlarge the ovaries up to 8 cm in diameter.

Massive oedema has been reported mostly in women in the reproductive age group. Typically, it is characterised by very marked oedema of the stroma, which also appears to be hyperplastic. The condition may be unilateral or bilateral. Occasionally, luteinisation of the affected stroma results in manifestations similar to those of the Stein-Leventhal syndrome or stromal hyperthecosis. Massive oedema may involve one or both ovaries, which can attain a diameter of 20 to 30 cm. The pathologist distinguishes the lesion from an oedematous fibroma or thecoma by finding follicular derivatives within the involved stroma.

Endometriotic cysts may be confused by cystic neoplasms of the ovary. Typically, they are associated with adhesions and other stigmata of that disorder. It must be remembered, however, that a variety of neoplasms, epithelial, stromal and mixed, may rarely arise from endometriotic tissue.

Preoperative and operative diagnosis of tumour type

Since it is only occasionally possible to establish the nature of an ovarian tumour preoperatively, the surgeon should always be aware of all the types of ovarian tumours and the age group, and be prepared to treat each of them specifically, before the abdomen is opened. Several generalisations may be helpful in making an appropriate differential diagnosis, preoperatively and at the time of exploration. The age of the patient is an important diagnostic clue. Less than one in 15 ovarian tumours in patients under the age of 45 will prove to be malignant, whereas the corresponding ratio in older women approaches one in three. The single most common ovarian tumour, the dermoid cyst, is encountered at all ages, as are most of the much rarer steroid hormone-producing tumours. Other ovarian neoplasms, in contrast, are largely restricted to various age periods. For example, the primitive germ-cell tumours are almost never encountered except in children and women under the age of 50 years. The malignant germ-cell tumour, which is seen on rare occasions in older women, is an adult form of cancer, usually of squamous cell type arising in a dermoid cyst. The common serous and mucinous cystadenomas are seen mostly in the reproductive age group. The borderline and invasive counterparts of these tumours, as well as endometrioid, clear cell and undifferentiated carcinomas, can also be encountered in young women, but become increasingly common in older patients, particularly those in the perimenopausal age group. The age distribution of metastatic carcinomas of the ovary parallels that of the various sites of origin of those tumours, most of which arise in the gastrointestinal tract. It must be emphasised that Krukenberg tumours of gastric origin are occasionally seen during the fourth decade and even rarely during the third.

The laterality of ovarian tumours is also a clue to their nature, as illustrated by the estimated frequency of bilateral involvement by various types (Table 2.2). A number of guidelines to diagnosis can be extracted from these figures. For example, the knowledge that ovarian cancer in general is bilateral in only about 25% of the cases, and that metastatic carcinomas, which account for approximately 8% of ovarian cancers, are bilateral in over two-thirds of the cases, leads to the deduction that bilateral ovarian cancer is metastatic, usually from the gastrointestinal tract, in about 20% of the cases. This conclusion indicates that an especially careful search should be made for a carcinoma elsewhere when bilateral ovarian cancer is encountered at surgery. Once the nature of a primary ovarian cancer has been established, knowledge of the frequency of bilaterality may also be helpful when the possibility

Table 2.2 Bilaterality of ovarian tumours

Type	Approximate %	Type	Approximate %
Metastatic carcinoma	70	Fibroma	8
Lymphoma	50	Brenner tumour	5
Gonadoblastoma	35	Mucinous cystadenoma	4
Serous carcinoma	33	Granulosa cell tumour	4
Serous borderline	25	Sertoli-Leydig cell tumour	4
Undifferentiated carcinoma	25	Clear cell carcinoma	3
Endometrioid carcinoma	12	Immature teratoma	< 1
Dermoid cyst	12	Endodermal sinus tumour	< 1
Mucinous carcinoma	10	Thecoma	< 1
Mucinous borderline	10	Malignant dermoid cyst	0
Serous cystadenoma	10		
Dysgerminoma	10		

of ovarian and uterine conservation to preserve fertility is being considered in a young patient. For example, all the primitive germ-cell tumours, except for dysgerminoma, are rarely bilateral, so that contralateral adenexectomy with hysterectomy does not improve the prognosis in stage IA cases. The appearance of the contralateral ovary in cases of immature teratoma deserves special comment because it contains a neoplasm in about 10% of the cases. The latter, however, is almost invariably benign and usually a dermoid cyst. Therefore, the presence of a tumour in a contralateral ovary does not always indicate that it is of the same nature as the neoplasm being primarily treated.

Several generalisations may be helpful with regard to the surgeon's appraisal of the gross features of an ovarian tumour at surgery. A hard consistency may reflect the desmoplastic stroma of a carcinoma, but may be related to benign proliferation of a fibromatous component of the tumour instead. Papillary and polypoid excrescences are compatible with borderline and benign neoplasia, respectively, and do not necessarily indicate invasive cancer. In many cases, the nature of an ovarian tumour by external observation or palpation cannot be assessed accurately. Thus, solid tumours may be benign or malignant, and a thin-walled cyst filled with clear fluid, although usually benign, may be a borderline or invasive tumour, even an undifferentiated carcinoma. The carcinoma in such cases may appear as one or a few polypoid masses or as a slight velvety thickening of the inner lining of the cyst, once it has been opened.

The role of the pathologist in the diagnosis and management of ovarian tumours

It is evident from the FIGO staging system for ovarian cancer that the pathologist plays a key role in staging as well as diagnosis. Optimally, the pathologist should be in the operating room and be appraised of the diagnostic and therapeutic problems as they unfold. After the specimen is excised, the pathologist should be informed of sites of adhesion or rupture, since careful microscopical examination of such areas may be vital to the decision whether or not to administer adjuvant therapy. Whenever it may prove helpful to the surgeon in decision making at the time of operation, a frozen section should be considered. Frozen sections of ovarian tumours are often difficult to interpret, with the degree of difficulty depending on the experience of the individual pathologist. The pathologist should never be pushed, therefore, to make a diagnosis if unsure. If any doubt exists about the malignant nature of the tumour, the surgeon should proceed as conservatively as possible with the option of reoperating at a later date once the diagnosis has been established on the basis of permanent sections. Ascitic fluid, or cell washings, if fluid is absent, should be presented to the pathologist for cytological examination, and an extensive omental biopsy is optimally performed for staging purposes. Any questionable area of extension of the tumour or implant should be biopsied. It is important to emphasise that as many biopsy specimens as feasible should be obtained. One or two samples are not always representative of what is going on in unsampled areas.

The pathologist has several responsibilities on receiving a specimen from a patient with ovarian cancer, including making an accurate diagnosis of the type of tumour and recording the quantity of malignant tissue within the entire specimen. Additionally, the neoplasm should be graded, and it should be determined whether the serosal surface has been violated by invasion. Areas of adhesion and rupture require special attention. Biopsy material which appears grossly negative should be extensively sampled for microscopical examination, especially if the presence or absence of tumour will influence the management of the patient. It is only through the close cooperation of the gynecologist and pathologist that an accurate assessment of the disease can be made and optimal management guaranteed.

REFERENCES

Aguirre P, Scully R E 1982 Malignant neuroectodermal tumor of the ovary. A distinctive form of monodermal teratoma. American Journal of Surgical Pathology (submitted)
Bullon A Jr, Arseneau K, Prat J, Young R H, Scully R E 1981 Tubular Krukenberg tumor: a problem in histopathologic diagnosis. American Journal of Surgical Pathology
Chalvardjian A, Scully R E 1973 Sclerosing stromal tumors of the ovary. Cancer 31: 664–670
Clement P B, Scully R E 1980 Large solitary luteinized follicle cyst of pregnancy and puerperium. A clinicopathological analysis of eight cases. American Journal of Surgical Pathology 4: 431–438
Dickersin G R, Kline I W, Scully R E 1981 Small cell carcinoma of the ovary with hypercalcemia. A report of eleven cases. Cancer (In press)
Fox H, Langley F A 1976 Tumours of the ovary. Year Book Medical Publishers, Chicago

Hart W R 1977 Ovarian epithelial tumors of borderline malignancy (Carcinomas of low malignant potential). Human Pathology 8: 541–549

Hart W R, Norris H J 1972 Borderline and malignant mucinous tumors of the ovary. Histologic criteria and clinical behavior. Cancer 31: 1031–1045

Kurman R J 1975 Personal communication

Kurman R J, Norris H J 1976a Endodermal sinus tumor of the ovary. A clinical and pathologic analysis of 71 cases. Cancer 38: 2404–2419

Kurman R J, Norris H J 1976b Embryonal carcinoma of the ovary. A clinicopathologic entity distinct from endodermal sinus tumor resembling embryonal carcinoma of the adult testis. Cancer 38: 2420–2433

Kurman R J, Norris H J 1977 Malignant germ cell tumors of the ovary. Human Pathology 8: 551–564

Kurman R J, Norris H J 1976c Malignant mixed germ cell tumors of the ovary. A clinical and pathologic analysis of 30 cases. Obstetrics and Gynecology 48: 579–589

Morris J McL, Scully R E 1958 Endocrine pathology of the ovary. C V Mosby, St Louis, 151 pp

Mostoufizadeh H, Scully R E 1980 Malignant tumors arising in endometriosis. Clinical Obstetrics and Gynecology 23: 951–963

Prat J, Bhan A K, Dickersin G R, Robboy S J, Scully R E 1982b Hepatoid yolk sac tumor of the ovary (endodermal sinus tumor with hepatoid differentiation). A light microscopial, ultrastructural and immunohistochemical study of seven cases. Cancer (Submitted)

Prat J, Scully R E 1981 Cellular fibromas and fibrosarcomas of the ovary: a comparative clinicopathologic analysis of 17 cases. Cancer 47: 2663–2670

Prat J, Young R G, Scully R E 1982a Ovarian Sertoli-Leydig cell tumors with heterologous elements. Cancer (Submitted)

Robboy S J, Norris H J, Scully R E 1975 Insular carcinoid primary in the ovary. A clinicopathologic analysis of 48 cases. Cancer 36: 404–418

Robboy S J, Scully R E 1980 Strumal carcinoid of the ovary: An analysis of 50 cases of a distinctiye tumor composed of thyroid tissue and carcinoid. Cancer 46: 2019–2034

Robboy S J, Scully R E, Norris H J 1974 Carcinoid metastatic to the ovary: a clinicopathological analysis of 35 cases. Cancer 33: 798–811

Robboy S J, Scully R E, Norris H J 1977 Primary trabecular carcinoid of the ovary. Obstetrics and Gynecology 49: 202–207

Rome R M, Fortune D W, Quinn M A, Brown J B 1981 Functioning ovarian tumors in postmenopausal women. Obstetrics and Gynecology 57: 705–710

Samanth K K, Black W C III, 1970 Benign ovarian stromal tumors associated with free peritoneal fluid. American Journal of Obstetrics and Gynecology 107: 538–545

Scully R E 1963 Germ cell tumors of the ovary. In: Meigs J V, Sturgis S H (eds) Progress in gynecology. Grune and Stratton, New York, vol 4, p 335–347

Scully R E 1968 Classification, pathology and biologic behavior of ovarian tumors. Meadowbrook Staff Journal 1: 148–163

Scully R E 1970 Recent progress in ovarian cancer. Human Pathology 1: 73–98

Scully R E 1977a Ovarian tumors. A review. American Journal of Pathology 87: 686–720

Scully R E 1977b Sex cord-stromal tumors. In: Blaustein A (ed) Pathology of the female genital tract. Springer-Verlag, New York, p 505–526

Scully R E 1979a Tumors of the ovary and maldeveloped gonads. Armed Forces Institute of Pathology, Washington, D.C.

Scully R E 1979b Ovarian tumors with endocrine manifestations. In:DeGroot L J et al (eds) Metabolic basis of endocrinology. Grune and Stratton, New York, ch 115, p 1473–1488

Scully R E 1981b Neoplasia associated with anomalous sexual development and abnormal sex chromosomes. Pediatric Adolescent Endocrinology 8: 203–217

Scully R E 1981a Pathology of the female genital tract after prenatal exposure to diethylstilbestrol. In: Developmental effects of diethylstilbestrol (DES) in pregnancy. A L Herbst, H A Bern (eds) Thieme-Stratton, New York, ch 3

Scully R E, Barlow J F 1967 'Mesonephroma' of ovary. Tumor of mullerian nature related to the endometrioid carcinoma. Cancer 29: 1405–1417

Serov S F, Scully R E 1972 Histological typing ovarian tumors. International Histological Classification of Tumors No. 9 World Health Organization, Geneva

Serov S F, Scully R E, Sobin L H 1973 Histological typing of ovarian tumours. International Histological Classification of Tumours no. 9. World Health Organization, 56 pp

Talerman A A 1972 A distinctive gonadal neoplasm related to gonadoblastoma. Cancer 30: 1219–1224

Taylor H B, Norris H J 1967 Lipid cell tumors of the ovary. Cancer 20: 1953–1962

Teilum G 1965 Classification of endodermal sinus tumour (mesoblastoma vitellinum) and so called 'embryonal carcinoma' of the ovary. Acta pathologica et microbiologica scandinavica 64: 407–429

Young R H, Carey R W, Robboy S J 1981 Breast carcinoma masquerading as primary ovarian neoplasm. Cancer 48: 210–212

Young R H, Prat J, Scully R E 1982a Ovarian Sertoli-Leydig cell tumors with heterologous elements (1) gastrointestinal epithelium and carcinoid. A clinicopathologic analysis of 36 cases. Cancer (submitted)

Young R H, Welch W R, Dickersin G R, Scully R E 1982b Ovarian sex cord tumor with annular tubules. Cancer (In press)

Zaloudek C J, Tavassoli F A, Norris H J 1981 Dysgerminoma with syncytiotrophoblastic giant cells. A histologically and clinically distinctive subtype of dysgerminoma. American Journal of Surgical Pathology 5: 361–367

3

Borderline ovarian carcinomas

Introduction

Certain ovarian tumours are on the histological borderline between benign ovarian cystadenomas and invasive ovarian cystadenocarcinomas. These borderline tumours are characterised by the absence of stromal invasion by the tumour cells but the presence of some characteristics indicative of malignancy. In certain instances, these tumours are associated with death from metastasis. Borderline tumours occur most frequently in women between the ages 20–40. Considering the age group affected, the most important aspect of these tumours is that the survival rate is nearly 100% when treated in their earliest stages, even by conservative unilateral salpingo-oophorectomy, which allows these women to retain their child-bearing capability.

In 1963, because of the high cure rate and the lack of histological evidence of invasion, the International Federation of Gynecologists and Obstetricians (FIGO) accepted this intermediate group of ovarian carcinomas as a separate entity, and designated them carcinomas of low malignant potential.' In 1973, the World Health Organisation's Histologic Classification of Ovarian Tumours Committee adopted the term 'borderline malignancies' to describe these tumours.

Although the survival rate for stage I borderline ovarian carcinomas approximates 100%, and is still markedly improved even when there is spread beyond the ovary, 50% of the cases in the advanced stages will eventually die of malignancy. Therefore, it is important to recognise these tumours as a distinct entity and to treat them promptly.

Diagnosis of borderline carcinomas

The borderline tumours are characterised by an unusual degree of epithelial cell proliferation but with no invasion of the adjacent stroma. Morphological features consist of epithelial cell stratification (usually three layers or less), increased mitotic activity, nuclear abnormalities, cytologically atypical cells and small cellular buds which may be formed by the proliferating cells which may detach from the primary tumour. When making the diagnosis, the pathologist should examine one block of tissue for every 1 to 2 cm of tumour. Histologically, they are most commonly serous or mucinous and very rarely demonstrate endometrioid or mesonephric characteristics. The diagnosis is made by evaluation of the primary tumour alone, without reference to clinical evidence (presence or absence) of distant metastasis. Metastasis from, or recurrence of these tumours retain the histological characteristics of the primary borderline tumour.

Stage and bilaterality

The incidence of spread beyond the ovary, the rate of bilaterality and the eventual cure rate are important considerations when determining the treatment for borderline ovarian tumours. Julian & Woodruff (1978) reported a 45% incidence (30/64) of extra-ovarian involvement in their series of serous borderline ovarian tumours. Of the 55 cases reported by Katzenstein et al (1978), 45% (25) had serous tumours that extended beyond the ovary at initial diagnosis. Bilaterality (stage IB) occurred in 40% of the 30 stage I serous borderline tumours reported by Katzenstein et al and in 26 (9/34) of the stage I serous borderline tumours in the Julian & Woodruff study. The incidence of extra-ovarian spread from mucinous borderline ovarian tumours is considerably less than that of the serous type, with less than 5% reported by Hart & Norris (1973).

Survival

Stage I borderline ovarian tumours

As seen in Table 3.1, the five-year actuarial survival rate for stage I borderline ovarian tumours ranges from 90–100%. At 10 years,

Table 3.1 Stage I borderline ovarian carcinoma; actuarial survival (5–20 years)

Authors	5 Years (%)	10 Years (%)	20 Years (%)
Hart & Norris 1973	98	96	–
Julian & Woodruff 1978	100	–	–
Katzenstein et al 1978	100	–	–
Aure et al stage IA 1971	96	94	78
stage IB	94	86	86
Kolstad et al 1977	90	–	–

the actuarial survival rate reported by Hart & Norris was still excellent at 96%. However, the survival rate reported by Aure for stage IA tumours at 10 years was 94%, and decreased to 86% at 10 years for stage IB tumours.

Of more concern is the 20-year actuarial survival rate for stage IA and IB borderline tumours reported by Aure of 78% and 86%, respectively. The results of Aure's study indicate that 14–22% of the patients with borderline ovarian tumours will die of their disease if followed for a considerable period of time. This report, if confirmed by other investigators, would indeed change the management of borderline ovarian tumours because conservative therapy would be inappropriate for a disease associated with a 14–22% mortality rate, even at 20 years. Since the entity of borderline ovarian tumours is a recently established category, there are no other reports of 20-year follow-up. However, as previously stated, Hart & Norris reported an actuarial survival rate for stage I borderline ovarian tumours of 96% at 10 years. Even Aure suggests caution as his retrospective analysis was based on a review of slides available from 1945–1964 before there was the actual borderline ovarian tumour entity and before sections were taken of every 1 to 2 cm of tumour. As Aure stated, 'It is necessary to bear in mind, however, that finding tumour infiltration (invasion) may depend on the number of sections taken' (Aure et al 1971).

The survival rate for stage I borderline ovarian carcinoma is excellent and is significantly better than that for a histologically similar invasive type of carcinoma confined to the ovary. Hart & Norris (1973) compared their stage I mucinous borderline ovarian tumours with their stage I invasive mucinous ovarian adenocarcinomas (Table 3.2). The 5-year and 10-year actuarial survival rates are considerably better for the borderline ovarian tumours, 98% and 96%, compared to the 5-year and 10-year survival rates of 66% and 59% for stage I invasive mucinous adenocarcinomas.

Table 3.2 Survival rates (5 & 10 years) with borderline and invasive ovarian mucinous carcinoma* (Hart & Norris 1973)

Histology	5 Year (%)	10 Year (%)
Borderline	98	96
Invasive	66	59

* Excludes patients lost to follow-up

Katzenstein et al (1978), reported 100% survival rate for 27 stage IA and IB patients with serous borderline ovarian carcinomas, 19 of whom received no treatment other than surgery (Table 3.3). Similarly, of the 25 patients with stage IA serous borderline ovarian tumours in the Julian & Woodruff (1978) study, 15% were treated by unilateral salpingo-oophorectomy; and the five-year survival rate was 100%. A five-year survival rate of 100% was also achieved in 10 patients treated by hysterectomy and bilateral salpingo-oophorectomy (one patient died of intercurrent disease).

Table 3.3 Survival rate with borderline serous carcinomas (Katzenstein et al 1978)

Stage	Patients	Survival NED* (%)	Received no adjuvant treatment
IA	15	100	11
IB	12	100	8
IIA	3	100	1
IIB	5	40	0
III	16	56	0

* NED = No evidence of disease

The first prospective, randomised study of borderline ovarian tumours is that reported by Kolstad et al (1977), who randomised patients with stage I borderline ovarian tumours to pelvic radiotherapy (5000 rads), or pelvic radiotherapy (3000 rads) plus intraperitoneal radioactive gold (100 millicuries). The five-year survival rates were 92.5% and 87.2%, respectively. The poor results with pelvic radiotherapy plus radioactive gold were caused by two deaths from complications. The overall survival rate from tumour-related deaths was quite excellent, however, with only one of 46 patients treated with pelvic radiotherapy (2.7%), and one of 37 patients (2.7%) treated with pelvic radiotherapy and radioactive gold, dead from their tumours. These low mortality rates were comparable to the 96 to 100% survival rates reported by Hart & Norris (1973), Julian & Woodruff, (1978), Katzenstein et al (1978), and Aure et al (1971).

71

Survival: stage II-IV borderline ovarian carcinomas

In the Katzenstein report (1978), no patient with borderline ovarian tumour confined to one or both ovaries had a recurrence or has died of tumour. Also, none of their patients with stage IIA (3) died of tumour. Of the 21 patients with stage IIB and stage III borderline ovarian tumours, 51% (11) were alive without evidence of disease. This percentage is considerably better than that reported for invasive carcinoma stages IIB and III (Table 3.3).

Better survival rates were reported by Julian & Woodruff (1978) for metastatic borderline ovarian carcinomas. Of their 30 patients with extra-ovarian involvement, stages II–IV, they achieved a corrected five-year survival rate of 85.2% (Table 3.4).

Table 3.4 Survival rate with borderline serous carcinomas of the ovary with extra-ovarian involvement (Julian & Woodruff 1978)

Stage	Patients	Corrected survival (%)
IIA	7	100
IIB	7	86
III	11	82
IV	5	80
	30	85

Treatment and conclusion

When a unilateral ovarian tumour is discovered in a young patient, a unilateral salpingo-oophorectomy should be performed and the tumour should be sent for a frozen section evaluation. If a frozen section diagnosis of a borderline ovarian tumour is made, and if careful evaluation of the other ovary, pelvis and upper abdomen demonstrates no evidence of malignancy, no further surgery should be performed. The specimen should then be evaluated by examining every 1–2 cm of tumour by permanent section evaluation to confirm the absence of invasion. In adults, not desiring further child bearing, total abdominal hysterectomy and bilateral salpingo-oophorectomy should be performed. Again, careful evaluation of the pelvis and upper abdomen including the diaphragm, omentum, retroperitoneal lymph nodes and cytological washings should be done.

Because of the near 100% survival rate in stage I borderline ovarian tumours, no adjuvant therapy for such lesions is required. This may change if other investigators can document the 14–22% mortality rate at 20 years of follow-up in stage I borderline ovarian tumours as reported by Aure et al (1971). Then, indeed, the use of adjuvant therapy as for invasive stage I tumours would be appropriate (see Ch. 5 Stage I ovarian carcinoma). For those patients with extra-ovarian involvement by borderline ovarian tumours, stages II–IV, treatment should be that for invasive carcinoma for the respective stages.

REFERENCES

Aure J C, Hoeg K, Kolstad P 1971 Clinical and histologic studies of ovarian carcinoma. Obstetrics and Gynecology 37: 1
Hart W R, Norris H J 1973 Borderline and malignant mucinous tumours of the ovary. Cancer 31: 1031
Julian C G, Woodruff J D 1978 The biologic behavior of low grade papillary serous carcinoma of the ovary. Obstetrics and Gynecology 40: 860
Katzenstein A L A, Mazur M T, Morgan T E, Kao M S 1978 Proliferative serous tumours of the ovary. American Journal of Surgical Pathology 2: 339
Kolstad P, Davy M, Hoeg K 1977 Individualized treatment of ovarian cancer. American Journal of Obstetrics and Gynecology 128: 617

4

Staging laparotomy in stage I and II ovarian malignancies

Introduction

The reasons for the poor survival rates of women with stage I ovarian malignancies, treated by either hysterectomy and bilateral salpingo-oophorectomy (67%), or hysterectomy and bilaterial salpingo-oophorectomy and postoperative radiation (60%) (Bagley et al 1972), remained enigmatic until the recent discovery of the sites of subclinical metastasis from stage I and II ovarian malignancies. Many of these areas of subclinical metastasis were never included within the treatment field for clinical stage I and II ovarian cancer, and therefore, poor survival rates resulted (Table 4.1).

Table 4.1 Ovarian adenocarcinoma; summary (from literature review) of 5-year survival rates (Bagley et al 1972)

FIGO stage	Surgery only	Surgery + radiotherapy	Surgery + chemotherapy
I	67% (32–78)	60% (40–71)	94%
IA	63% (46–78)	66% (53–70)	–
IB	70% (59–80)	50% (36–70)	–
IC		43% (40–50)	–

Historically, four reports led to the now formalised staging laparotomy in early ovarian cancer. In 1940, Pemberton advocated that, 'When an operation for cancer of the ovary is done it would be wise to remove the omentum, regardless of whether or not gross metastasis can be seen in it, because it is so often effected and may be the source of recurrence later.' It was approximately 35 years later, however, that the first prospective study was done which documented the incidence of subclinical metastasis in normal appearing omenta in stage I ovarian cancer (Knapp & Friedman 1974). In 1956, Keettel & Elkin reported that peritoneal washings (injection and collection of fluid from the pelvis) were cytologically positive for free-floating malignant cells in a significant number of patients with clinical stage IA ovarian cancer. Even with the descriptions in the 1940s and 1950s of these two sites of subclinical metastasis, no further evaluation for other sites of failure in treating stage I and II ovarian cancer was carried out for nearly 20 years.

The impetus for more formalised staging laparotomy of patients with localised ovarian cancer was prompted by the report of Bagley et al (1973). Five stage I and II ovarian cancer patients, referred for postoperative therapy, underwent laparoscopic examination of the peritoneal cavity and were found to have unsuspected diaphragmatic metastasis. This series was subsequently updated by Rosenoff et al (1975) to 16 stage I or II ovarian cancer patients, 44% of whom had diaphragmatic metastasis (Table 4.2).

Table 4.2 Peritoneoscopy in ovarian carcinoma; frequency of diaphragmatic metastasis (Rosenoff et al 1975)

Laparotomy stage	Patients	Diaphragmatic metastasis
I or II (localised)	16	7 (44%)
III or IV (advanced)	33	23 (70%)
All stages	49	30 (61%)

This incidence of diaphragmatic metastasis seemed to explain the previously inexplicable 30–40% mortality rate from early ovarian cancer. However, we subsequently evaluated 31 consecutive patients with stage I and II ovarian cancer and had only one patient (3.2%) with unsuspected diaphragmatic metastasis (Piver et at 1978). Clearly, the diaphragm was an important source of failure to survive from early ovarian cancer, but did not by itself explain the poor overall survival rates. Notwithstanding our reported low incidence of diaphragmatic metastasis, the report in 1975 by Rosenoff et al (Table 4.2) demonstrated that the diaphragm may be one of the most common sites of metastasis in all ovarian cancer stages. It is now well documented that the diaphragm, para-aortic and pelvic lymph nodes, omentum, and malignant peritoneal washings are five sites of subclinical metastasis in presumed stage I and II ovarian cancer.

Diaphragmatic metastasis

After Bagley's initial report (1972) of diaphragmatic metatasis, other investigators evaluated the incidence of such metastasis from early stage ovarian cancer. As seen in Table 4.3, 15.7% of the 70 patients with stage I and II ovarian cancer had metastasis to the diaphragm; 11.3% for stage I and 23% for stage II (Rosenoff et al 1975, Piver et al 1978, Spinelli et al 1976, Delgado et al 1977). The pumping action of the diaphragm that occurs with each respiration, causes free-floating cancer cells to move from the pelvis through the peritoneal cavity and into the diaphragmatic lymphatics. The right subdiaphragmatic area is primarily involved. The left subdiaphragmatic area is rarely involved without first metastasis to the right, because the splenorenal ligament on the left acts as a mechanical barrier to free-floating cancer cells on the left side of the peritoneal cavity.

Table 4.3 Ovarian cancer stage I & II; diaphragmatic metastases (Piver et al 1978)

Author	Patients	Incidence (%)
Rosenoff	16	43.7 (7)*
Spinelli	13	23.0 (3)
Delgado	10	0.0 (0)
Piver	31	3.2 (1)
Total	70	15.7 (11)
Total stage I	44	11.3(5)
Total stage II	26	23.0 (6)

* Number of patients

Para-aortic nodal metastasis

Knapp & Friedman (1974) reported the first prospective study which evaluated the incidence of unsuspected para-aortic lymph node metastasis from stage I ovarian cancer. They performed para-aortic lymphadenectomies on 24 women with stage I ovarian cancer and discovered 12.5% had para-aortic lymph node metastasis (two patients were excluded because of histological evidence of left supraclavicular lymph node metastasis). Musumeci et al (1977a) initially reported 24 patients with stage I ovarian cancer and one stage II patient who underwent para-aortic lymph node

Table 4.4. Ovarian cancer stage I & II; aortic lymph node metastases (Piver et al 1978)

Author	Patients	Incidence (%)
Musumeci	28	7.0 (2)*
Knapp	24	12.5 (3)
Delgado	10	20.0 (2)
Piver	5	0.0 (0)
Total	67	10.4 (7)
Total stage I	57	12.2 (7)
Total stage II	10	10.0 (1)

* Number of patients

biopsy. This study was subsequently updated to 28 stage I patients. Two (7%) of the 28 patients had metastasis to the para-aortic lymph nodes (Musumeci et al 1977b). Both had stage IA tumours. As outlined in Table 4.4, the incidence of para-aortic lymph node metastasis from stage I and II ovarian cancer for 67 patients is 10.4%. For stage I, the incidence is 12.2% and for stage II, the incidence is 10% (Knapp & Friedman 1974, Delgado et al 1977, Musumeci et al 1977a, 1977b, Piver et al 1978).

Omental metastasis

The first prospective study which evaluated the incidence of subclinical omental metastasis from stage I and II ovarian cancer was completed by Knapp & Friedman (1974), 35 years after Pemberton's report on the significance of removing the omentum in ovarian malignancies. Knapp & Friedman performed a partial omentectomy by resecting the omentum from the transverse colon in 21 patients with stage I ovarian cancer, and only 4.7% (1) had

Table 4.5 Ovarian cancer stage I & II; omental metastases (Piver et al 1978)

Author	Patients	Incidence (%)
Knapp	21	4.7 (1)*
Delgado	10	0.0
Piver	5	0.0
Total	36	2.7 (1)
Total stage I	27	3.7 (1)
Total stage II	9	0.0

* Number of patients

omental metastasis (one patient was excluded due to metastasis of the left supraclavicular lymph node). Of the 36 patients (Table 4.5) who had prospective evaluation for omental metastasis for stage I or II ovarian cancer, only 2.7% were found to have subclinical omental metastasis. This included a 3.7% incidence for stage I and a 0% incidence for stage II (Knapp & Friedman 1974, Delgado et al 1977, Piver et al 1978).

Malignant peritoneal cytology

Keetel & Elkin initially reported the finding of positive peritoneal washings in 1956 and in 1974 this study was updated to a total of 44 patients with stage IA ovarian cancer (intact capsule). Sixteen patients (36%) had positive peritoneal washings (Keettel et al 1974). We evaluated 31 consecutive stage I or II ovarian carcinoma patients, and performed pelvic and paracolic washings. (Fig. 4.1) Free-floating cancer cells were found in 25.8%, including 30.4% for stage I and 12.5% for stage II. Of the 87 patients

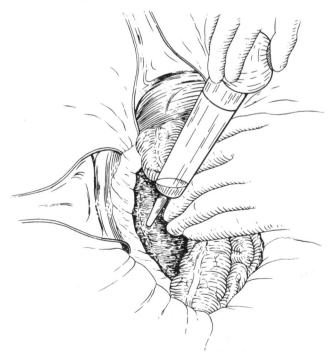

Fig. 4.1 Peritoneal washings from the right pericolic space

Table 4.6 Ovarian cancer stage I & II; malignant cytological washings (Piver et al 1978)

Author	Patients	Incidence (%)
Keettel	44	36.3 (16)*
Creasman	10	10.0 (1)
Morton	2	50.0 (1)
Piver	31	25.8 (8)
Total	87	29.8 (26)
Total stage I	79	31.6 (25)
Total stage II	8	12.5 (1)

* Number of patients

reported (Table 4.6), 29.8% had positive cytological washings, including 31.6% for stage I and 12.5% for stage II (Morton et al 1961, Creasman & Rutledge 1971, Keettel et al 1974, Piver et al 1978).

Pelvic node metastasis

Knapp & Friedman (1974), in their prospective evaluation of stage I ovarian cancer patients, performed selected pelvic lymph node biopsies of the external iliac, internal iliac and obturator lymph nodes in nine patients, none of which contained metastasis. In the reports by Musumeci (1977a, 1977b) of 28 stage I ovarian cancer patients, 10.6% (3) were found to have biopsy-proven metastasis to the pelvic lymph nodes; including two patients with metastasis to the common iliac lymph nodes, and one patient with metastasis to the external iliac lymph nodes. In these two series, 8.1% (3/37) had pelvic node metastasis.

The incidence of stage I ovarian cancer metastasis

It is clear from Table 4.7 that the incidence of subclinical metastasis from stage I ovarian cancer: diaphragm 11%, omentum 3%, para-aortic lymph nodes 10%, pelvic lymph nodes 8% and malignant peritoneal washings 33%, accounts for the poor survival rate by surgery alone in stage I ovarian cancer. Moreover, any therapy that will increase survival rates in early stage ovarian cancer will have to be directed toward these five sites of early metastasis.

Table 4.7 Stage I ovarian adenocarcinoma; incidence of subclinical metastases (Piver et al 1978)

Site	Patients	Incidence %
Diaphragm	44	11
Omentum	27	3
Para-aortic lymph node	58	10
Pelvic lymph node	37	8
Malignant peritoneal washings	79	33

Staging laparotomy: Ovarian Cancer Study Group

The Ovarian Cancer Study Group did a prospective evaluation on the incidence of subclinical metastasis in stage I and II ovarian cancer patients (Young et al 1979). All patients were referred to the four participating institutions within four weeks of surgery and underwent restaging laparatomy. In all 50 patients, the referring physician had stated there was no postoperative evidence of residual cancer. As seen in Table 4.8, 5% were found to have diaphragmatic metastasis, 7% omental metastasis, 15% para-aortic lymph node metastasis and 12% pelvic lymph node metastasis; a 24% overall incidence rate of unsuspected residual cancer.

Table 4.8 Restaging laparotomy in early ovarian cancer; incidence of previously unsuspected residual cancer in 50 patients with stage I & II disease. (Young et al 1979)

Site	%
Diaphragm	5
Omentum	7
Para-aortic lymph nodes	15
Pelvic lymph nodes	12
Other abdominal sites	8
Unsuspected residual cancer	24

Surgical staging procedures

It is now clear that the diaphragm, omentum, para-aortic lymph nodes, pelvic lymph nodes and malignant peritoneal cytological washings are sites of subclinical or small metastasis from early ovarian cancer and that they account for the 30–40% mortality rate in stage I ovarian malignancies. Therefore, when a clinically localised ovarian tumour is discovered at the time of pelvic laparotomy, histological confirmation should be obtained by frozen section evaluation. Then, the incision should be extended above the umbilicus for careful abdominal evaluation, and 100 cc of saline should be injected into the pelvis and the right paracolic and left paracolic spaces, respectively. This fluid is then sent for cytological evaluation. The diaphragmatic nodules should be biopsied by laparascopic biopsy forceps. There is minimal or no morbidity associated with biopsy of diaphragmatic metastasis. Random biopsies of a normal-appearing diaphragm are not advocated. The omentum should be inspected, and even if no evidence of metastasis is seen, an omentectomy should be carried out by removing the omentum from the inferior portion of the transverse colon. Any enlarged para-aortic lymph node along the course of the aorta and vena cava should be biopsied. Similarly, any enlarged pelvic lymph node should be sent for histological evaluation. Finally, the large and/or small bowel should be carefully evaluated.

Summary and conclusions

It is clear that early sites of metastasis from clinically localised ovarian malignancies occur in the diaphragm, omentum, para-aortic and pelvic lymph nodes, and malignant peritoneal cytological washings. What is not clear is how to use and transfer this knowledge, which should increase survival rates, to surgeons who discover most of the clinically localised ovarian cancer, but who are not trained in para-aortic or pelvic lymph node surgery. Clearly, most gynaecologists are well trained in removing the primary ovarian tumour and would have no difficulty in biopsing a raised tumour in the subdiaphragmatic area, resecting the omentum from the transverse colon, and obtaining cytological washings from the pelvis and paracolic spaces. They would be uncomfortable, however, in completing the staging procedure as related to removal of para-aortic, vena caval and pelvic lymph nodes. Therefore, now that the five primary sites of subclinical metastases are well documented, the next most important discovery is an effective therapy that will eradicate small or subclinical metastasis to them, after a surgeon has removed what is clinically a localised ovarian cancer.

REFERENCES

Bagley C M Jr, Young R C, Canellow G P et al 1972 Treatment of ovarian carcinoma: possibilities for progress. New England Journal of Medicine 288: 856

Bagley C M Jr, Young R C, Schein P S et al 1973 Ovarian carcinoma metastatic to the diaphragm frequently undiagnosed at laparotomy. A preliminary report. American Journal of Obstetrics & Gynecology 116: 397

Creasman W T, Rutledge F 1971 The prognostic value of peritoneal cytology in gynecologic malignant disease. American Journal of Obstetrics and Gynecology. 110: 773

Delgado G, Chun B, Caglar H 1977 Para-aortic lymphadenectomy in gynecologic malignancies confined to the pelvis. Obstetrics and Gynecology 50: 418

Keettel W C, Elkins H B 1956 Experience with radioactive gold in the treatment of ovarian carcinoma. American Journal of Obstetrics and Gynecology 71: 553

Keettel W C, Pixley E E, Buschsbaum H J 1974 Experience with peritoneal cytology in the management of gynecologic malignancies. American Journal of Obstetrics and Gynecology 120: 174

Knapp R C, Friedman E A 1974 Aortic lymph node metastases in early ovarian cancer. American Journal of Obstetrics & Gynecology 119: 1013

Morton D G, Moore J G, Chang N 1961 The clinical value of peritoneal lavage for cytologic evaluation. American Journal of Obstetrics and Gynecology 81: 1115

Musumeci R, Banfi A, Bolis G et al 1977a Lymphangiography in patients with ovarian epithelial cancer. Cancer 40: 1444

Musumeci R, Banfi A, DePalo G et al 1977b Lymphangiography in patients with ovarian epithelial cancer. Proceedings of the Sixth International Congress of Lymphology Prague (personal communication)

Pemberton F A 1940 Carcinoma of the ovary. American Journal of Obstetrics and Gynecology 40: 751

Piver M S, Barlow J J, Lele S B 1978 Incidence of subclinical metastasis in stage I and II ovarian carcinoma. Obstetrics and Gynecology 52: 1

Rosenoff S H, DeVita V T Jr, Hubbard S et al 1975 Peritoneoscopy in the staging and follow-up of ovarian cancer. Seminars in Oncology 2: 223

Spinelli P, Luini A, Pizzetti P et at 1976 Laparoscopy in staging and restaging of 95 patients with ovarian carcinoma. Tumori 62: 493

Young R C, Warton J T, Decker D G, Piver M S, Edwards B, McGuire W F 1979 Staging laparotomy in early ovarian cancer. Proceedings American Association of Cancer Research and American Society of Clinical Oncology 20: 399

5

The treatment of stage I and II ovarian carcinomas. Radioactive chromic phosphate (^{32}P), radioactive gold (^{198}Au), whole abdominal irradiation and systemic chemotherapy

Introduction

Survival rates for stage I ovarian cancer patients treated by surgery alone, or by surgery in combination with radiation therapy have not been satisfactory. Bagley et al (1972) and Fuks (1977) have reviewed the literature on survival rates independently, and their results are nearly identical. Bagley et al reported a 67% survival rate for stage I patients treated with surgery alone, and a 60% survival rate for those treated with a combination of surgery and radiation therapy. Fuks reported 70% and 58% survival rates, respectively, for stage I ovarian cancer patients treated with surgery alone, and with a combination of surgery and radiation therapy, primarily pelvic irradiation (Table 5.1). These poor results,

Table 5.1 Five year survival rates in stage I, II, III ovarian carcinoma 1960–1975 (Fuks 1977)

Stage	Surgery alone No.	%	Surgery + irradiation No.	%
I	270/389	70	411/707	58
II	22/103	21	221/693	32
III	14/280	5	105/1020	10

at the earliest stage of ovarian cancer, indicate the need for a therapeutic approach which can effect a significantly higher cure rate.

Even in presumed localised ovarian cancer (stages I and II) treatment must be directed to the areas of occult or subclinical metastasis: the diaphragm, omentum, para-aortic lymph nodes, pelvic lymph nodes and free-floating cancer cells. To date, there are three rational methods for eradicating subclinical metastasis in each of these areas: (1) intraperitoneal chromic phosphate or radioactive gold; (2) whole abdominal irradiation using large open fields or strip irradiation to the whole abdomen, and (3) systemic chemotherapy.

Intraperitoneal chromic phosphate [^{32}P] and radioactive gold [^{198}Au] for stage I ovarian carcinomas

Although no prospective, randomised clinical trials on the use of ^{32}P and ^{198}Au in treating stage I ovarian cancer patients have been reported, the results of a retrospective analysis of their use provides a reasonable expectation that clinical trials will result in over 90% cure rates (Rosenshein et al 1979), a vast improvement over conventional therapies.

Muller (1963) reported that 150 millicuries of ^{198}Au diluted in 400 ml of saline, delivered approximately 4000 rads to the peritoneal serosa, 6000 rads to the omentum and an average of 7000 rads to the retroperitoneal lymph nodes. However, these results have not been documented by other investigators. The dose delivered to the retroperitoneal, para-aortic and pelvic lymph nodes is considered to be less than the reported 7000 rads. Moreover, the exact dose of radiation from ^{32}P or ^{198}Au needed to eradicate small clusters of tumour cells is not known. Notwithstanding this lack of dose response data, the most important information is what can be achieved clinically that will result in cure rates of over 90%.

Most institutions that use radioactive isotopes use intraperitoneal ^{32}P and have discontinued the use of intraperitoneal ^{198}Au. This is due in part to the significant complications which have resulted from the use of intraperitoneal ^{198}Au that are not commonly seen with intraperitoneal ^{32}P. These complications are believed to be due to the differences in characteristics of the two substances (Table 5.2). ^{32}P is a pure beta irradiation emitter,

Table 5.2 Characteristics of radioactive chromic phosphate and gold

Characteristic	^{32}P	^{198}Au
Physical	Colloidal suspension	Colloid
Half-life	14.5 days	2.7 days
Maximum energy	960 ku	1700 ku
Radioactive emission	Beta particles	Beta particles + gamma rays
Maximum tissue penetration	4.6 mm	4 mm
Dose	15 mCi	150 mCi

whereas ^{198}Au, in addition to emitting beta irradiation, also emits gamma rays. The shorter half-life of ^{198}Au of 2.7 days, compared to 14.5 days for ^{32}P, results in irradiation of the tissues at a higher rate, which may be associated with the higher incidence of complications. ^{32}P is preferred to ^{198}Au because its high beta energy results in greater tissue penetration; its long half-life makes it easier to order and use compared to the short half-life for ^{198}Au, which requires almost immediate use and its pure beta particle emissions are not harmful to hospital personnel and patient isolation is not required. The gamma rays from ^{198}Au are harmful to exposed individuals and isolation of the patient for approximately one week is required. The patient treated with ^{32}P can be discharged the day following treatment.

^{32}P emits its irradiation in the form of electrons (beta particles). During the partial disintegration of the radioactive isotopes, they emit ionising irradiation which can destroy small clusters of tumour cells. The important considerations for the use of radioactive isotopes is that they are absorbed by the peritoneal surface, including the diaphragmatic lymphatics and that they are then absorbed into the mediastinal lymphatics, the right thoracic trunk, the right subclavian vein and finally, that they enter the general circulation, leaving small deposits in the liver, spleen, kidney, and lung.

Methods of installation of ^{32}P

Catheter placement and pretherapy peritoneogram

A polyethylene or silastic fine catheter may be left in the peritoneal cavity at the time of surgery. If not placed at that time, a number 14 gauge angiocatheter is inserted into the peritoneal cavity, under local anesthesia, approximately one week after surgery. A peritoneogram, using approximately 30 cc of renographin-60, is performed as a precaution to prevent the inadvertent injection

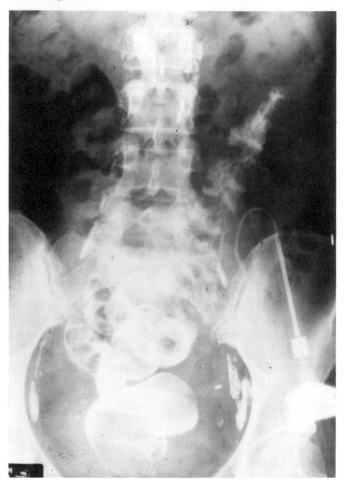

Fig. 5.1 Inadvertent injection of dye into the colon at time of attempted peritoneogram

of the ^{32}P into the intestine (Fig. 5.1). Figure 5.2 demonstrates a normal peritoneogram with good distribution of the dye above the liver and throughout the peritoneal cavity. The main contra-indication to the use of ^{32}P in stage I ovarian cancer would be the presence of multiple adhesions that would prevent its even distribution in the peritoneal cavity.

Injection of intraperitoneal ^{32}P

As stated above, poor results will occur using ^{32}P if there is uneven

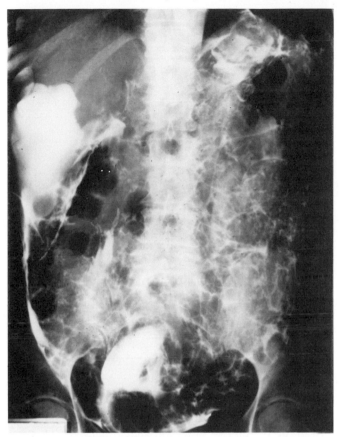

Fig. 5.2 Normal dispersion of dye at time of peritoneogram

distribution throughout the peritoneal cavity. Rosenshein et al (1978) used female adult rhesus monkeys to demonstrate that using small volumes of fluid to instil radioactive isotopes into the peritoneal cavity fails to produce the even distribution required and results in inadequate treatment of many areas of the peritoneal cavity. Therefore, it is important to use sufficiently large volumes of solutions to aid in the uniform distribution of ^{32}P. Using large quantities of solutions also takes advantage of the pumping action of the diaphragm to distribute the ^{32}P throughout the peritoneal cavity.

The procedure begins with the injection of 400 cc of saline into the peritoneal cavity to create a hydroperitoneum. This is followed by the bolus injection of 15 millicuries of ^{32}P. An additional 600 cc

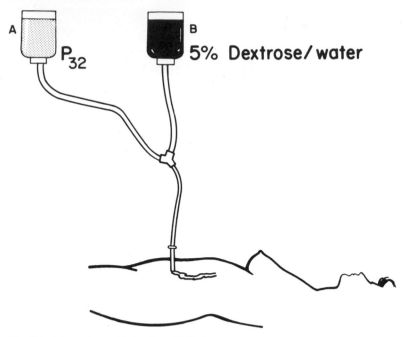

Fig. 5.3 Intraperitoneal injection of 5% dextrose in water followed by chromic phosphate [^{32}P] and 5% dextrose in water

of saline is then injected intraperitoneally to aid in the uniform distribution of ^{32}P (Fig. 5.3). Latex gloves are worn during the injection of ^{32}P, and all materials, including the tubing, are disposed of in the manner of any radioactive material. The injection site is sutured to prevent leakage of ^{32}P.

Following injection, the patient is turned every 15 minutes for approximately two hours in five different positions to ensure even distribution: head down supine, right side, prone, left side and head elevated. To evaluate the distribution of ^{32}P, an abdominal scan is performed the day following injection. Although ^{32}P is a pure beta emitter, Bremsstrahlung X-rays (less than 1% of total energy) are emitted which allow for the production of adequate scans. Figure 5.4 demonstrates uniform distribution of the intraperitoneally injected ^{32}P throughout the peritoneal cavity.

Complications

We reported 74 patients with stage I, II, and III ovarian cancers treated with ^{32}P or ^{198}Au using the technique described (Table

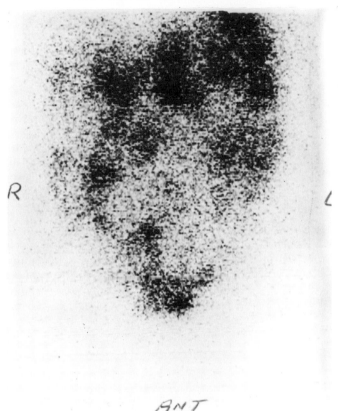

Fig. 5.4 Post-injection scan demonstrating uniform distribution of the intraperitoneally injected ^{32}P

Table 5.3 Complications of intraperitoneal radio colloids (Piver 1972)

Complications	Number		%
None	63		85.1
Abdominal pain	3		
Ileus	1	Minor	13.5
Fever	5		
Subcutaneous injection	1	Major	
Intestinal obstruction	1		1.4
	74		100

5.3).Intestinal obstruction was the only major complication that occurred (1.4%). This was relieved by intestinal tube decompression (Piver 1972). Many patients who received ^{198}Au also received external radiation therapy which may, in part, have contributed

Table 5.4 Major complications of intraperitoneal chromic phosphate (^{32}P) in stage I ovarian cancer

Authors	Patients	Major complications	%
Alderman et al 1977	21	1 Intestinal obstruction	4.7
Hester & White 1969	33	None	0.0
Clark et al 1973	28	None	0.0
	82	1	1.2

to the higher complication rate associated with ^{198}Au. Keettel et al (1976) reported a 4.3% incidence of major complications, primarily related to intestinal obstruction, fistula and peritonitis, in 220 patients treated by intraperitoneal ^{198}Au. Decker et al (1973) reported an 11% incidence of small bowel obstruction in 142 patients treated with intraperitoneal ^{198}Au. As seen in Table 5.4, the use of ^{32}P in 82 women with stage I ovarian cancer resulted in only one major complication (1.2%), an intestinal obstruction relieved by lyses of adhesions (Hester & White 1969, Clark et al 1973, Alderman et al 1977).

Survival after intraperitoneal ^{32}P and ^{198}Au

Primarily using intraperitoneal ^{32}P, we have reported a 94.4% survival rate (Table 5.5) without evidence of recurrence from three to 13 years after surgery (Piver 1972). Combining our data with other institutions using ^{32}P for stage I ovarian cancer, the survival rate, without evidence of recurrence, was 92.7% (Hester & White 1969, Clark et al 1973). This is considerably better than the 67% and 70% survival rates reported by the use of surgery alone (Bagley et al 1972, Fuks 1977).

Table 5.5 Survival in stage I ovarian cancer after use of intraperitoneal chromic phosphate [^{32}P]

Authors	Patients	Survival* No.	%
Piver 1972	18	17	94.4
Clark et al 1973	28	26	92.8
Hester & White 1969	9	8	88.8
	55	51	92.7

* Without evidence of recurrence, 3–13 years after surgery

The survival rate after the use of intraperitoneal [198]Au for stage I ovarian cancers has ranged from 50% in small series to as high as 94.3% in larger series. Buchsbaum et al (1975) reported a relative survival of 94.3% in 56 patients treated for stage I ovarian adenocarcinoma with 150 millicuries of [198]Au, and Moore & Langley (1967) reported a 90% survival with the use of intraperitoneal [198]Au in 10 patients with stage I ovarian cancer. Decker et al (1973) treated 56 patients with intraperitoneal [198]Au for stage I ovarian cancer and reported only a 73.2% survival rate. However, when they compared their 25 patients with stage IC (rupture of the capsule), who presumably had free-floating cancer cells treated by intraperitoneal [198]Au, to their 22 stage IC patients treated by surgery alone, the five-year survival rates were 80 to 43%, respectively.

External irradiation or systemic ohcmotherapy: stage I and II ovarian malignancies

Stage I

'High radiation doses to the entire peritoneal surfaces are not feasible due to limited tolerance of some of the abdominal organs such as the liver, kidneys, intestine, stomach and bone marrow, however, even with the appropriate shielding of vital viscera, insuring that tolerance is not exceeded, whole abdominal irradiation has been poorly tolerated by most patients. Furthermore, the radiation dose levels required for tumour sterilization in ovarian cancer is essentially unknown...(radiation doses) are not supported by data on dose response curves and determinations of local recurrences for each dose level. In fact such data do not even exist for ovarian carcinoma.' (Fuks 1977)

This pessimistic view of the use of radiotherapy in the management of the ovarian cancer patient has recently had an increasing number of supporters.

Historically, patients who received postoperative irradiation for ovarian carcinoma, received either pelvic irradiation or open field irradiation to the entire abdomen. It is clear from the pattern of metastasis of ovarian carcinoma that very few patients would benefit from radiation directed only to the pelvis. Open field whole abdominal irradiation is limited to a dose of approximately 3000 rads in six to eight weeks because of severe intestinal reactions and patient tolerance.

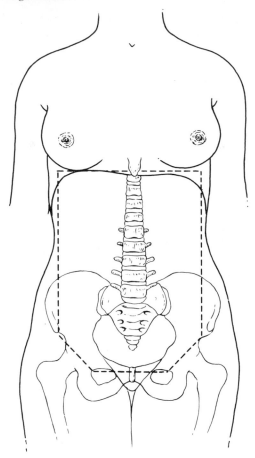

Fig. 5.5 Open field whole abdominal radiation

Using whole abdominal irradiation, the entire pelvis and abdomen are included from the mid obturator foramen of the pelvis to the dome of the diaphragm during each treatment (Fig. 5.5). A daily fraction of approximately 160 rads is given for five days each week. The maximum dose to the upper abdomen is approximately 3000 rads, with the kidney and liver shielded after 2000 to 2500 rads to prevent radiation nephritis and radiation hepatitis, respectively. An additional 2000 rads may be delivered to the pelvis for a maximum dose of 5000–5500 rads. Therefore, dose limitations of approximately 3000 rads to the intestines and 2000 and 2500 rads to the liver and kidney in six to eight weeks should be effective in sterilising small, residual or subclinical disease but would not result in a significant eradication of tumours greater than 1 mm in diameter. The problem is complicated further by the recent finding of diaphragmatic metastasis, primarily of the right dia-phragm, in ovarian cancer patients. This area is shielded at the time when the liver and kidney are shielded, and therefore, derives limited benefit from the radiation. Within the foreseeable future, a solution to the intolerance of the small intestines, liver and kidney areas is not apparent.

A larger biological effect therefore was required if irradiation was to play a major role in the treatment of ovarian cancer. Patient tolerance to irradiation is influenced by the total dose delivered, the volume of tissue irradiated and the duration of each treatment. Therefore, it was theorised that the same dose to a smaller area, given for a shorter period of time, should have a much greater biological effect. With this in mind, the moving strip technique was developed.

The moving strip technique, with cobalt-60, is used in some institutions to overcome the two main disadvantages of open field irradiation to the whole abdomen by irradiating smaller areas to lessen intestinal reactions over a shorter period of time, to obtain a larger biological effect. The abdomen is divided into 2.5 cm strips. Each strip is irradiated four times anteriorly and four times posteriorly for a total dose of approximately 2800 rads, in eight treatments, within 10 calendar days. In the moving strip tech-nique, on day one, a 2.5 cm strip is irradiated both anteriorly and posteriorly and treatment fields are increased by one strip every two days until 10 cm (four strips) have been included within the

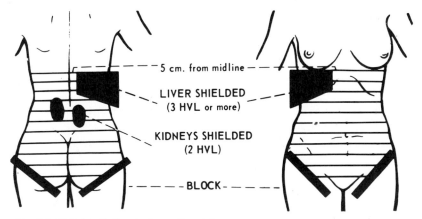

Fig. 5.6 Strip irradiation to the entire abdomen

treatment field. Once this 10 cm area has been treated, it receives no further irradiation. Then a new 2.5 cm strip is started the next day until the whole abdomen has been irradiated (Fig. 5.6). The very small areas irradiated should allow for a greatly improved intestinal tolerance. Because the dose is administered in a much shorter time, its biological effect is greater even when the total dose is the same as open field whole abdominal irradiation. According to present concepts of time/dose relationships, a dose of 3000 rads in 10 days is equivalent to 4500 rads in six weeks (Friedman et al 1970). Unfortunately, the one randomised prospective study did not show a significant difference in survival rates between the two methods — i.e., open field whole abdominal irradiation vs. strip irradiation, although there was less morbidity with the moving strip technique (Fazekas & Maier 1974).

Smith and coauthors (1975) compared whole abdominal irradiation by the moving strip technique to the use of melphalan chemotherapy as adjuvant treatment in early ovarian carcinomas.

Table 5.6 Selection of treatment regimes in randomised trial by Smith et al 1975

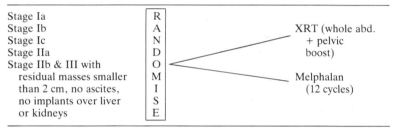

As seen in Table 5.6, patients with stages IA, IB, IC, IIA or IIB and III disease, with residual masses smaller than 2 cm, no ascites, or no implants on the liver or kidneys were randomised to receive either whole abdominal irradiation or melphalan chemotherapy. Unfortunately, there were significantly more patients with stage IIB disease, and therefore, more volume of tumour in the radiotherapy group (32) compared to the melphalan group (22). However, there was no difference in survival rates when all stages were combined. The actuarial survival rate for patients with stage I ovarian carcinoma was approximately 90% for those treated by melphalan alone, compared to 85% for those receiving whole abdominal irradiation (Fig. 5.7). Moreover, there was significantly more morbidity in the group treated with whole abdominal irradiation than the group treated by melphalan. This is a preliminary report with only a few patients at risk at five years. Subse-

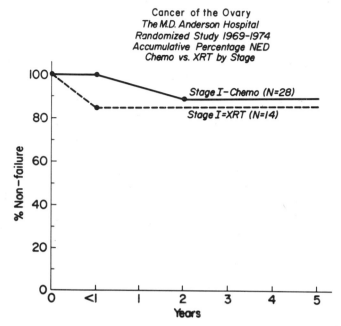

Fig. 5.7 Survival rates after whole abdominal radiation or chemotherapy in stage I ovarian malignancies

quent updating of the survival and morbidity data is required before the clinical usefulness of this report can be fully assessed.

The Gynecologic Oncology Group recently reported a prospective study which compared pelvic irradiation to no therapy, or melphalan chemotherapy, for patients with stage I ovarian carcinoma (Hreshchyshyn et al 1980). Patients were randomised to no treatment, pelvic irradiation (5000 rads in five to six weeks), or melphalan (0.2 mg/kg/day for five days every four weeks for 18 months) (See Table 5.7). Follow-up ranged from four to 83 months, with a median of 36 months. As seen in Table 5.8, even with short follow-up for many patients, melphalan was superior

Table 5.7 GOG stage I ovarian adenocarcinoma study* (Hreshchyshyn et al 1980)

Randomisation after surgery	Patients
I No adjuvant therapy	29
II Pelvic irradiation: 5000 rads/5–6 weeks	23
III Chemotherapy: Melphalan 1 mg/kg monthly X 18	34

* Follow-up 4–83 months. Median 36 months. Not staged.
 Not stratified for stage (IA, IB), grade, histology.

Table 5.8 GOG stage I ovarian adenocarcinoma study: recurrence rate following various treatment regimes (Hreshchyshyn et al 1980)

Treatment	Patients	Recurrence
No therapy	29	17% (5)
Pelvic irradiation	23	30% (7)
Melphalan	34	6%* (2)
Total	86	16% (14)

* $P = <0.05$

to no treatment or pelvic irradiation. Only 6% of the patients treated by melphalan have developed recurrences compared to a 30% recurrence rate for those patients receiving pelvic irradiation and a 17% recurrence rate for those receiving no therapy. Some patients have been followed for only a few months and very few are at risk at five years. However, it is clear that no therapy or only pelvic irradiation are not effective for most patients with stage I ovarian carcinomas. Longer follow-up of the patients treated with melphalan is required before this can be advocated as standard adjuvant therapy for patients with stage I disease.

Stage II

The data on therapy of stage II ovarian carcinoma patients is sparse because most patients with ovarian cancer are diagnosed after the malignancy has spread beyond the pelvis (stages III and IV), or less commonly, when the tumour is clinically limited to the ovary. In a recent report of 24 patients with stage II ovarian carcinoma receiving postoperative pelvic irradiation (5–6000 rads), only 38% survived five years (Wallner et al 1977). If indeed there is a significant incidence of diaphragmatic metastasis, free-floating cancer cells, para-aortic nodal metastasis and omental metastasis in stage II ovarian cancer, the use of pelvic irradiation would result in a 60%, or greater, number of patients developing recurrences.

In Fuks' review (1977), the five-year survival rates for patients undergoing surgery alone for stage II ovarian carcinoma averaged 21% (range 0–33%) compared to 32% (range 13–60%) for patients treated by surgery plus irradiation. Using the megavoltage technique, Fuks reported a five-year actuarial survival rate of 51%

Table 5.9 Ovarian carcinoma: survival rates at M.D. Anderson Hospital and Tumor Institute (Smith & Rutledge 1975).

Type of treatment	Stage I %	Stage II %	Stage III %	Stage IV %	Total %
Abdomen and pelvic irradiation	76	35	22	0	37
Abdomen only irradiation	58	21	6	0	26
Radioisotopes	78	19	9	0	25
Pelvis only irradiation	80	18	5	0	19

in 71 patients with stage II ovarian carcinoma, with no significant difference in survival between stages IIA or IIB. Similarly, as seen in Table 5.9, the survival rate in stage II patients treated at the M.D. Anderson Hospital and Tumour Institute by the whole abdominal irradiation, plus additional pelvic irradiation, was only 35% and even lower (21%) for those patients receiving whole abdominal irradiation without the addition of the pelvic irradiation (Smith & Rutledge 1975). It is clear that these poor survival rates by irradiation alone, in what is thought to be limited disease, are not satisfactory. To date, there are no prospective studies using other modalities of therapy that demonstrate significantly improved survival rates over these presented above.

Summary

Although no prospective study has documented the efficacy of intraperitoneal radioactive isotopes as adjuvant therapy over surgery alone for stage I ovarian carcinoma, a retrospective analysis of the low complication (1.2%) and the high cure rate (92.7%) of ^{32}P in stage I ovarian carcinoma speaks for its continued use until, and unless, improved therapy can be documented. Whole abdominal irradiation by the moving strip technique may indeed result in cure rates of the same order as ^{32}P (>90%), but the morbidity will be significantly higher. The two prospective studies reported on the use of melphalan as adjuvant therapy in early ovarian carcinoma must await longer follow-up before this can be adjudged a superior adjuvant therapy. Finally, treatment of stage II ovarian cancer remains enigmatic, but may require pelvic irradiation to the local disease, followed by adjuvant chemotherapy as advocated for stage I ovarian carcinomas.

REFERENCES

Alderman S J, Dillon T F, Krummerman M S et al 1977 Postoperative use of radioactive phosphorous in stage I ovarian carcinoma. Obstetrics and Gynecology 49: 659

Bagley C M, Young R C, Canellow G P et al 1972 Treatment of ovarian carcinoma: possibilities for progress. New England Journal of Medicine 288: 856

Buchsbaum H J, Keettel W C, Latovrette H B 1975 The use of radioisotopes as adjunct therapy of localized ovarian cancer. Seminars in Oncology 2: 247

Clark D G C, Hilaria B, Roussis C, Brunschaig A 1973 The role of radiation therapy (including isotopes) in treatment of cancer of the ovary (results of 614 patients treated at Memorial Hospital New York, New York). Clinical cancer. Grune & Stratton, New York, vol. 5, p 227–235

Decker D G, Webb M J, Holbrook M A 1973 Radiogold treatment of epithelial cancer of the ovary. American Journal of Obstetrics and Gynecology 115: 751

Fazekas V T, Maier V G 1974 Irradiation of ovarian carcinomas. A prospective comparison of the open field and moving strip techniques. American Journal of Roentgenology Radiation Therapy Nuclear Medicine 120: 118

Friedman A B, Benninghoss D L, Alexander L L et al 1970 Total abdominal irradiation using Cobalt-60 moving strip technique. American Journal of Roentgenology Radiation Therapy Nuclear Medicine 108: 172

Fuks A 1977 The role of radiation therapy in the management of ovarian carcinoma. Israel Journal of Medical Science 13: 815

Hester L L, White L 1969 Radioactive colloidal chromic phosphate in the treatment of ovarian malignancies. American Journal of Obstetrics and Gynecology 103: 911

Hreshchyshyn M M, Park R C, Blessing J A et al 1980 The role of adjuvant therapy in stage I ovarian cancer. American Journal of Obstetrics and Gynecology 103: 911

Keettel W C, Fox M R, Longnecker D A, Latourette H B 1966 Prophylactic use of radioactive gold in the treatment of primary ovarian cancer. American Journal of Obstetrics and Gynecology 94: 766

Moore D W, Langley H 1967 Routine use of radiogold following operation for ovarian cancer. American Journal of Obstetrics and Gynecology 98: 624

Muller J H 1963 Curative aim and results of routine intraperitoneal radiocolloid administration in the treatment of ovarian cancer. American Journal of Roentgenology, Radiation Therapy, Nuclear Medicine 89: 533

Piver M S 1972 Radioactive colloids in the treatment of stage I ovarian cancer. Obstetrics and Gynecology 40: 42

Rosenshein N B, Blake D, McIntyre P A, et al 1978 The effect of volume on the distribution of substances instilled into the peritoneal cavity. Gynecology and Oncology 6: 106

Rosenshein N B, Leichner P K, Vogelsang G 1979 Radiocolloids in treatment of ovarian cancer. Obstetrics and Gynecology Surgery 34: 708

Smith J P, Rutledge F N 1975 Current status of therapy for ovarian cancer. In: Meigs J V, Storgis S H (eds) Progress in cancer. Grune and Stratton, New York, vol. 6

Smith J P, Rutledge F N, Delclos L 1975 Results of chemotherapy as adjunct to surgery in patients with localized ovarian cancer. Seminars in Oncology 2: 277

Wallner P E, Brady L W, Lues G C, Nuss R C 1977 Postoperative pelvic irradiation of stage II ovarian carcinoma. International Journal of Radiation Oncology Biology Physics 2: 281

6

First line chemotherapy and debulking surgery for stage III and IV ovarian adenocarcinoma

Single agent chemotherapy (Table 6.1)

Alkylating agents are standard therapy for patients with advanced ovarian adenocarcinoma. One of the initial reports demonstrating their effectiveness was from the M D Anderson Hospital & Tumor Institute in Houston, Texas describing their initial experience from 1956–1960. Of seven women with advanced ovarian adenocarcinoma treated with the chemotherapeutic agent melphalan (L-phenylalanine mustard), six had 'objective responses' (Samuels et al 1962). In the next update (Burns et al 1963) of their series, 93 patients with advanced ovarian adenocarcinoma were treated with melphalan; and 54.8% (51) had a partial response, greater than 50% reduction in tumour size. This extremely high response rate helped establish melphalan as one of the drugs of choice for advanced ovarian adenocarcinoma. At that same time, equally good response rates were reported for the other available alkylating agents: chlorambucil, cyclophosphamide and triethylene-thiophosphoramide.

To this point, melphalan and other alkylating agents had been used strictly as palliative therapy. In the next M D Anderson Hospital & Tumor Institute report in 1966, 213 women were treated with melphalan. The authors reported that 13 patients, 'had such unusually good response that laparotomy was performed even to determine if inoperable tumour had become removable or to evaluate the need for additional drug therapy. In each of the 13 patients, no tumour was found and chemotherapy was discontinued.' Melphalan was discontinued in the 13 women and only two had recurrence at the time of the report (Rutledge & Burns 1966). This important study established that single agent chemotherapy

Table 6.1 Active single agent chemotherapy in ovarian adenocarcinoma

Drug	Dose	Method of administration	Response rate	Major toxicity
1. Melphalan (Alkeran, L-phenylalanine mustard)	0.2 mg/kg/day × 5 q 4 wks	orally	20–50%	Mylosuppression nausea & vomiting
2. Chlorambucil (Leukeran)	0.2 mg/kg/day	orally	20–50%	Mylosuppression
3. Cyclophosphamide (Cytoxan, ENDOXAN)	3.0 mg/kg/day	orally	20–50%	Mylosuppression
	10 mg/kg/day × 5 q 4 wks	i.v.		haemorrhagic cystitis alopecia
4. Triethylenethiophosphoramide (THIO-TEPA)	0.2 mg/kg/day × 5 q 4 wks	i.v.	20–50%	Mylosuppression nausea & vomiting
5. Cis-Dichlorodiamine platinum II (Cis-platinum)	60–75 mg/m² q 3 wks	i.v.	20–35%	Nephrotoxicity hearing loss & tinnitus nausea & vomiting mylosuppression
6. Doxorubicin (Adriamycin)	60–90 mg/m² q 3 wks	i.v.	20–35%	Congestive heart failure alopecia stomatitis nausea & vomiting mylosuppression
7. Hexamethylmelamine (HXM)	8 mg/kg/day	orally	20–35%	Nausea & vomiting peripheral neuropathy mylosuppression
8. Methotrexate (Amethopterane) a. Citrovorum Calcium	0.5–1.0 g/m² q 4 wks 6–16 mg/m² q 6 hrs × 12	i.v. i.m.	15–25%	Stomatitis mylosuppression hepatotoxicity
9. 5-Fluorouracil (5-FU)	15 mg/kg/day × 5 q 4 wks	i.v.	15–25%	Mylosuppression nausea & vomiting diarrhoea alopecia

q = every

First line chemotherapy and debulking surgery

Table 6.2 Melphalan in advanced ovarian adenocarcinoma; response rates at the M.D. Anderson Hospital and Tumor Institute 1960–1969 (Smith & Rutledge 1970)

Courses	Patients	Total %	Complete %	Partial %	None %
≧ 3	494	47	20	27	53
< 3	91	0	0	0	100
Total	585	39	17	22	61

Table 6.3 Early reports of response rate to alkylating agents in ovarian adenocarcinoma

Drug	No. of pts.	Response	Authors	Year
Melphalan	585	39%	Smith & Rutledge	1970
Chlorambucil	280	50%	Masterson & Nelson	1965
Thio-tepa	144	64%	Wallach et al	1965
Cyclophosphamide	104	37%	Decker et al	1967

with melphalan could totally eradicate ovarian adenocarcinoma that was not removed surgically and actually lead to cure in a small percentage of such women. Finally, their series was updated to the end of 1969. They reported on 585 women treated with melphalan for advanced ovarian adenocarcinoma (Smith & Rutledge 1970). As seen in Table 6.2, the response rate had decreased from their earlier optimistic reports to a total response of only 39%, and a complete response rate* of only 17%. Many of the early reports (Table 6.3) of overall response rates using single alkylating agents were also quite high (Smith & Rutledge 1970, Masterson & Nelson 1965, Wallach et al 1965, Decker et al 1967).

Single agent chemotherapy: effect of complete response rate on ultimate survival

Our experience with single agent melphalan in 111 women with stage III or IV ovarian adenocarcinoma was inauspicious, with less than 20% responding and only 10.8% with complete responses (Piver et al 1978). The complete responders, however, had a meaningful increase in survival (median 19 months), compared to

---

* Throughout this book, a complete response to chemotherapy is defined as the complete disappearance of all clinical and roentgenographic evidence of malignancy lasting a minimum of one month, whereas a partial response is 50–99% decrease in measurable tumour.

Table 6.4 Melphalan in advanced ovarian adenocarcinoma, response and survival rates at Roswell Park Memorial Institute 1971–1975 (Piver et al 1978)

Response	%	(no. of patients)	Median survival (months)	Statistical difference
Complete	10.8	(12)	19.0	
Partial*	9.0	(10)	11.2	$P < 0.01$
No change*	28.8	(32)	10.7	$P < 0.01$
Progression	51.4	(57)	2.9	$P < 0.001$
Total	100.0	(111)		

* Partial & no change vs. progression $P < 0.001$

only 2.9 months for patients with progression of their disease ($P<0.001$). This survival was also significantly better than the less than one-year survival for those with partial responses, or no change in their tumour size ($P<0.01$). See Table 6.4. As seen in Figure 6.1, this was also evident in the study by Young et al (1974) in patients with stage III and IV ovarian adenocarcinoma treated with either melphalan or cyclophosphamide. Only those patients achieving a complete clinical response had a significant prolongation of survival. There were no differences in survival for those patients having a partial response or no response to chemotherapy. Therefore, it became apparent that meaningful responses and increased length of survival resulted only from complete responses to chemotherapy. Although some of the smaller, earlier series using melphalan reported quite high overall response rates, and

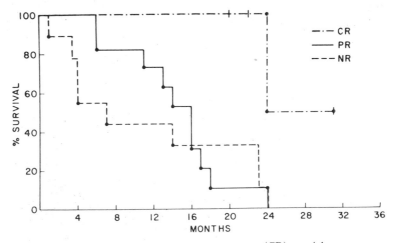

Fig. 6.1 Duration of survival after complete response (CR), partial response (PR), or no response (NR) to chemotherapy

Table 6.5 Responses to melphalan in cases of advanced ovarian carcinoma (Piver et al 1978)

Authors	Patients (no.)	Response Complete (%)	Total (%)
Smith	585	17.0	39.8
Brodovsky	114	17.0	26.0
Piver	111	10.8	19.8
Smith	50	20.0	42.0
Smith	33	12.0	24.0
Frick	28	0.0	21.4
Young	26	19.0	61.0
Rossoff	24	8.3	12.5
de Palo	20	10.0	20.0
Young	14	14.2	64.2
	1005	15.5	35.0

even high complete response rates, it can be seen in Table 6.5 that of 1005 patients treated with melphalan, the overall response rate was 35% with only 15.5% complete responses (Frick et al 1968, Smith & Rutledge 1970, Smith 1972, Smith et al 1972, Young et al 1974, 1976, DePalo et al 1975, Rossoff et al 1976, Brodovsky et al 1977, Piver et al 1978).

Although activity against ovarian adenocarcinoma by the anti-metabolites 5-fluorouracil and methotrexate had been reported, it was the important report of Wiltshaw & Kroner (1976), demonstrating a 26% response rate to cis-diaminodichloroplatinum (cis-platinum) as second-line chemotherapy in patients who had failed on initial first-line single alkylating agent chemotherapy, which led eventually to a significant improvement in overall responses in ovarian adenocarcinoma patients. At the same time, Bonadonna and his coworkers (1975) reported that the antibiotic agent adriamycin was effective in ovarian adenocarcinoma, with five of 17 patients responding. Hexamethylmelamine, which is structurally closely related to the alkylating agent triethylmelamine, but may not be an alkylating agent, has been shown to be active as a first-line therapy in advanced ovarian adenocarcinoma. Wharton et al (1979) reported a 31.7% response rate and a 14.8% complete response rate in 54 advanced ovarian adenocarcinoma patients treated with hexamethylmelamine. Therefore, it is clear that there are now a number of effective single agents against advanced ovarian adenocarcinoma, including the alkylating agents (melphalan, cyclophosphamide, chlorambucil, triethylenethiophosphoramide), as well as hexamethylmelamine, cis-diaminodichloroplatinum, adriamycin, 5-fluorouracil and methotrexate; that their overall response rates are comparable; and that complete response rates may be too low to significantly improve survival rates.

Melphalan chemotherapy vs. combination chemotherapy

The rationale for using combination chemotherapy is that agents with different mechanisms of action attack the cancer cell at different metabolic sites. In the first five prospective studies comparing melphalan to combination chemotherapy, approximately 50% responded to combination chemotherapy, while only 33% responded to melphalan (Frick et al 1968, Smith 1972, Smith et al 1972, Young et al 1976, Brodovsky et al 1977). However, the important number, the complete response rate, was only 25% for the combinations and 17% for melphalan (Table 6.6). The most active of these combinations, prior to the use of cis-platinum, was HEXACAF (hexamethylmelamine, cyclophosphamide, methotrexate and 5-fluorouracil). Comparing HEXACAF to single agent chemotherapy with melphalan, Young and coauthors (1978) updated their series, and reported a 75% (30/40) overall response rate to the combination chemotherapy compared to 54% for melphalan. The complete response rate was 33% for the combination chemotherapy and 16% for melphalan. Neijt et al (1980) used

Table 6.6 Comparison of response rates to Melphalan or combination chemotherapy (Piver et al 1978)

Combination	Response with combination			Response with melphalan		
	No. of patients	Complete (%)	Total (%)	No. of patients	Complete (%)	Total (%)
ACFUCY	49	28.6	53.1	49	18.4	34.7
ACFUCY	47	30.0	45.0	50	20.0	42.0
HC	32	25.0	53.0	33	12.0	24.0
HEXACAF	24	33.0	79.0	26	19.0	61.0
CMF	110	19.0	41.0	114	17.0	26.0
	262	24.8	48.8	272	17.2	33.7

ACFUCY = Actinomycin-D, 5-fluorouracil, cyclophosphamide
HC = Hexamethylmelamine, cyclophosphamide
HEXACAF = Hexamethylmelamine, cyclophosphamide, methotrexate, 5-fluorouracil
CMF = cyclophosphamide, methotrexate, 5-fluorouracil

HEXACAF in 23 previously untreated patients with advanced ovarian adenocarcinoma and achieved a 52% response rate, with only 22% complete responders. These complete response rates are not significantly better than single agent chemotherapy.

Highly active combination chemotherapy (Table 6.7)

Again, the important study of Wiltshaw & Kroner (1976), demonstrating that one of four patients will respond to cis-platinum as second-line chemotherapy, led many investigators to use cis-platinum as first-line chemotherapy in combination with the other active agents. Vogl et al (1979) using hexamethylmelamine, adriamycin, and cis-platinum (HAD) in 18 patients as second-line chemotherapy, achieved the outstanding response rate of 67%. This was significantly better than the 26% response rate reported by Wiltshaw & Kroner, using cis-platinum as second-line chemotherapy and was considerably better than the majority of reports documenting a 5–10% response rate for any second-line chemotherapy. Because of this unusually high response rate using HAD as second-line chemotherapy, the same authors used HAD plus cyclophosphamide in a four drug regimen, CHAD, as initial che-

Table 6.7 Highly active combination chemotherapy in ovarian adenocarcinoma

Combination	Dose	Dose		Response Total	Response Complete
CHAD				90.4%	47.6%
Cyclophosphamide	600 mg/m^2 Day 1		i.v.		
Hexamethylmelamine	150 mg/m^2 Days 8–21		p.o.		
Adriamycin	25 mg/m^2 Day 1		i.v.		
cis-Platinum	50 mg/m^2 Day 1		i.v.		
PAC				68.5%	37%
cis-Platinum	50 mg/m^2		i.v.		
Adriamycin	50 mg/m^2		i.v.		
Cyclophosphamide	750 mg/m^2		i.v.		
HEXACAF				75%	33%
Hexamethylmelamine	150 mg/m^2 Days 1–14		p.o.		
Cyclophosphamide	150 mg/m^2 Days 1–14		p.o.		
Amethopterane (Methotrexate)	40 mg/m^2 Days 1 + 8		i.v.		
Fluorouracil (5-FU)	600 mg/m^2 Days 1 + 8		i.v.		
MECY				67%	48%
Methotrexate	750 mg/m^2 Day 1		i.v.		
Cyclophosphamide	250 mg/m^2 1 Day X 5		i.v.		

motherapy. They reported the unusually high response rate to CHAD of 90.4% in 21 patients with previously untreated ovarian adenocarcinoma and, moreover, 47.6% had complete responses. Using a similar combination of cis-platinum, adriamycin and cyclophosphamide, but without hexamethylmelamine, as primary therapy in advanced ovarian adenocarcinoma, Ehrlich and co-authors (1979) reported an overall response rate of 68.5%, with a complete response rate of 37%. Using high-dose methotrexate and cyclophosphamide in previously untreated advanced ovarian adenocarcinoma patients, Barlow et al (1980) achieved an overall response rate of 68%, with a complete response rate of 48%.

Improved survival by debulking surgery and combination chemotherapy

At this point, the role of surgery in conjunction with adjuvant chemotherapy was unknown. Day & Smith (1975) reported on 388 patients with stage III ovarian adenocarcinoma who were evaluated for survival in relation to the size of residual disease after initial surgery. In these 388 patients, 27% survived five years when there was no residual cancer prior to initiation of chemotherapy or radiotherapy and 35% survived five years when the residual disease was less than 1 cm prior to initiation of adjuvant therapy. However, only 2% of the remaining 323 patients with residual disease greater than 1 cm survived five years. The improved survival with small residual cancer was also noted in the study by Griffiths (1975). For their stage II or III ovarian adenocarcinoma patients, the mean survival ranged from 39 months for no residual cancer to only 11 months for residual cancer measuring greater than 1.5 cm. There were no survivors past 26 months with residual cancer greater than 1.5 cm. (Table 6.8 a & b).

Therefore, it was evident that patients achieving a complete clinical response to chemotherapy and that patients with small residual tumor (0–2 cm), had significantly improved survival. However, the relationship between complete response and size of disease was still not apparent. This relationship became apparent in two recent reports. The complete response rate to melphalan or HEXACAF in patients who had residual cancer of less than 2 cm was 53%. It was 100% for the patients receiving HEXACAF and only 18% for melphalan (Young et al 1978). This is compared to a complete response rate of 15% for melphalan and 15% for HEX-

Table 6.8a Survival dependent on amount of residual disease: stage III ovarian carcinoma (Day & Smith 1975)

Residual tumour	Patients	Survival 5 years
0	34	27%
1 cm	31	35%
1.1 cm–2 cm	24	0%
2.1 cm–6 cm	95	0%
> 6 cm	172	5%
Unknown	32	0%
Total	388	

Table 6.8b Mean survival (months) dependent on size of residual ovarian carcinoma: 102 patients FIGO stages II & III (Griffiths 1975)

Size of residual cancer	Mean survival (months)*
None	39
0–0.5 cm	29
0.6–1.5 cm	18
> 1.5 cm	11

* No survivors past 26 months whose residual cancer was 1.5 cm

Table 6.9 Complete response dependent on size of residual cancer (Young et al 1978)

Chemotherapy	Complete Response Rate	
	<2 cm Residual (19)	>2 cm Residual (58)
Melphalan or HEXACAF	53%	15%
HEXACAF	100%	15%
Melphalan	18%	15%

( ) = Number of patients

ACAF for residual disease greater than 2 cm (Table 6.9). In a similar study on the relationship between complete response and the size of residual tumour, patients who had non-palpable disease at initiation of chemotherapy (most likely less than 2 cm), had a complete response rate of 91%, compared to a complete response rate of only 4% in patients with palpable disease (most likely greater than 2 cm) prior to initiation of chemotherapy (Parker et al 1980).

Summary and conclusions

It is clear that debulking surgery which reduces ovarian malignancies to aggregates of 2 cm or less is associated with an increased complete response rate to postoperative chemotherapy. Moreover, complete responses are associated with significant increase in survival compared to partial responses or no responses. Finally, the more recent chemotherapy combinations, including the active single agents against ovarian adenocarcinoma, are associated not only with significantly higher overall response rate but more importantly with an increase in complete responses. These highly active combinations are too new to know the long-term effect on survival.

REFERENCES

Barlow J J, Piver M S 1977 Single agent vs combination chemotherapy in the treatment of ovarian cancer. Obstetrics and Gynecology 49: 609–611
Barlow J J, Piver M S, Lele S B 1980 High dose methotrexate with rescue plus cyclophosphamide as initial chemotherapy in ovarian adenocarcinoma. Cancer 46: 1333
Bonadonna G, Berretta G, Tancini G et al 1975 Adriamycin studies at the National Cancer Institute, Milan. Cancer Chemotherapy Reports 6: 231–245
Brodovsky H S, Temkin N, Sears M 1977 Melphalan versus cyclophosphamide, methotrexate and 5-fluorouracil (CMF) in women with ovarian cancer. Proceedings of American Association of Cancer Research and American Society of Clinical Oncology 18: 308
Burns B C, Rutledge F, Gallagher H S 1963 Phenylalanine mustard in the palliative management of carcinoma of the ovary. Obstetrics and Gynecology 22: 30–37
Day T G, Smith J P 1975 Diagnosis and staging of ovarian carcinoma. Seminars in Oncology 2: 217–222
Decker D G, Mussey E, Malkasian G D, et al 1967 Adjuvant therapy for advanced ovarian malignancy. American Journal of Obstetrics and Gynecology 97: 171
dePalo G M, Delena M, DiRe F, et al 1975 Melphalan versus adriamycin in the treatment of advanced ovarian carcinoma of the ovary. Surgical Gynecology and Obstetrics 141: 899–902
Ehrlich C E, Einhorn L, William S S, Morgan J 1979 Chemotherapy for stage III–IV epithelial ovarian cancer with cis-diaminodichlorplatinum II, adriamycin, and cyclophosphamide: A preliminary report. Cancer Treatment Reports 63: 281
Frick H C, Tretter P, Tretter W et al 1968 Disseminated carcinoma of the ovary treated by L-phenylalanine mustard. Cancer 21: 508–513
Griffiths C T 1975 Surgical resection of tumor bulk in the primary treatment of ovarian carcinoma. Symposium on ovarian carcinoma, National Cancer Institute Monograph 42: 101–104
Masterson J G, Nelson J H Jr 1965 The role of chemotherapy in the treatment of gynecologic malignancy. American Journal of Obstetrics and Gynecology 93: 1102
Neijt J P, VanLindert A, Vendric C et al 1980 Treatment of advanced ovarian carcinoma with a combination of hexamethylmelamine, cyclophosphamide, methotrexate and 5-fluorouracil in patients with and without previous treatment. Cancer Treatment Reports 64: 323

Parker L M, Griffiths C T, Yankee R, Canellos G P et al 1980 Combination chemotherapy with adriamycin-cyclophosphamide for advanced ovarian carcinoma. Cancer 46: 669

Piver M S, Barlow J J, Yazigi R, Blumenson L 1978 Melphalan chemotherapy in advanced ovarian carcinoma. Obstetrics and Gynecology 51: 352

Rossoff A H, Drukker B H, Talley R W et.al 1976 Randomized evaluation of chlorambucil and melphalan in advanced ovarian cancer. Proceedings of American Society of Clinical Oncology 17: 300

Rutledge F, Burns B C 1966 Chemotherapy for advanced ovarian cancer. American Journal of Obstetrics and Gynecology 96: 761–772

Samuels M L, Howe C D, MacDonald E J 1962 Alkylating agents in the treatment of patients with advanced cancer of ovary, carcinoma of the uterine cervix, endometrium and ovary. Year Book Medical Publishers, Chicago, p 329–338

Smith J P 1972 Personal communication

Smith J P, Rutledge F 1970 Chemotherapy in the treatment of cancer of the ovary. American Journal of Obstetrics and Gynecology 107: 691–702

Smith J P, Rutledge F, Warton J T 1972 Chemotherapy of ovarian cancer. Cancer 30: 1565–1571

Vogl S E, Bernzweig M, Kaplan B et al 1979 CHAD and HAD regimens in advanced ovarian cancer: combination chemotherapy including cyclophosphamide, hexamethylmelamine, adriamycin and cis-dichlorodiaminoplatinum II. Cancer Treatment Reports 63: 311

Wallach R C, Kabakow B, Blinick G et al 1965 Thiotepa chemotherapy for ovarian carcinoma: Influence of remission and toxicity on survival. Obstetrics and Gynecology 25: 475

Wiltshaw E, Kroner T 1976 Phase II study of cis-dichlorodiaminoplatinum II in advanced adenocarcinoma of the ovary. Cancer Treatment Reports 60: 55

Wharton J T, Rutledge F, Smith J, et al 1979 Hexamethylmelamine: An evaluation of its role in the treatment of ovarian cancer. American Journal of Obstetrics and Gynecology 133: 833

Young R C, Chabner B A, Hubbard S B et al 1978 Advanced ovarian adenocarcinoma. New England Journal of Medicine 299: 1261

Young R C, DeVita V T, Chabner B A 1974 Chemotherapy of advanced ovarian carcinoma: A prospective comparison of phenylalanine mustard and high dose cyclophosphamide. Gynecologic Oncology 2: 489–497

Young R C, DeVita V T, Chabner B A 1976 A prospective trial of melphalan and combination chemotherapy in advanced ovarian cancer. Proceedings of American Association of Cancer Research & American Society of Clinical Oncology 17: 279

7

Second-line and third-line chemotherapy in metastatic ovarian adenocarcinoma

Second-line chemotherapy

Clearly, all ovarian adenocarcinomas are not responsive to initial chemotherapy and many that are initially sensitive to chemotherapy eventually demonstrate evidence of regrowth. Second-line chemotherapy is therefore required. Moreover, some patients are candidates for third and even fourth and fifth-line trials, although very few patients who failed on first or second-line chemotherapy respond.

Until recently, there was very little physicians could do after a patient had progression of ovarian malignancy on first-line chemotherapy. Stanhope et al (1977) reported only a 6% response rate in 347 patients receiving second-line chemotherapy (Table 7.1). However, the 26% response rate to second-line chemotherapy with cis-diaminodichloroplatinum (cis-platinum) reported by Wilt-

Table 7.1 Response to second-line chemotherapy in a advanced ovarian adenocarcinoma (Stanhope et al 1977)

Drugs	No.	%
ACFUCY*	9/145	6.2
Melphalan	8/71	11.3
5-Fluorouracil	1/46	2.2
Adriamycin	0/27	0
Cyclophosphamide & Hexamethylmelamine	1/9	11.1
Hexamethylmelamine	1/12	8.3
Thiotepa	1/4	25.0
Other	0/33	0.0
Total	21/347	6.0

* Actinomycin-D, 5-fluorouracil, cyclophosphamide

shaw & Kroner (1976) was significantly better than previous reports and has led to improved therapy for patients with progression of their ovarian malignancy after initial chemotherapy. Other new agents reported at that time included adriamycin and hexamethylmelamine. These agents were moderately effective as single agent, first-line chemotherapy but only a small percentage responded to these agents as second-line chemotherapy and very few (0.6%) achieved a complete clinical response (Table 7.2). (de Palo et al 1975, Wiltshaw & Kroner 1976, Bolis et al 1978, Bolis et al 1979, Bonomi 1979, Johnson et al 1979, Stehman et al 1979, Thigpen et al 1979).

Table 7.2 Second-line single agent chemotherapy

Drug	Patients	Response CR + PR (%)	Complete Response (%)	Authors
Cis-platinum	34	26	3	Wiltshaw & Kroner 1976
Cis-platinum	34	29	6	Thigpen et al 1979
Cis-platinum	12	25	0	Stehman et al 1979
Hexamethylmelamine	34	6	0	Bolis et al 1979
Hexamethylmelamine	21	18	0	Johnson et al 1978
Hexamethylmelamine	16	25	6	Bonomi et al 1979
Adriamycin	38	8	0	Bolis et al 1978
Adriamycin	27	0	0	Stanhope et al 1977
Adriamycin	6	16	0	de Palo et al 1975

Although the overall response to hexamethylmelamine, cis-platinum and adriamycin as second-line chemotherapy was low when used separately, the combination of these agents has been highly effective. Vogl et al (1979) reported a 63% response rate in 22 patients treated with the combination of hexamethylmelamine, adriamycin and cis-platinum (HAD) as second-line chemotherapy in patients who had failed on single alkylating agent therapy. Moreover, 18% had a complete clinical response. Kane and co-authors (1979) used the same three drug combination, but added cyclophosphamide (CHAP)* as second-line chemotherapy. They treated 35 women and achieved a 49% response rate, including 20% complete responses (Table 7.3). There has been some question of the efficacy of adriamycin in these regimens. In their preliminary report, Davis et al (1980) used only hexamethylmelamine and cis-platinum, but without adriamycin as second-line chemotherapy. They reported a 57% response rate in 22 patients, including 20% complete responses. We treated 20 women with the

Table 7.3 Second-line combination chemotherapy

Combination	Patients	Response CR + PR (%)	Complete Response (%)	Authors
I. CHAP Cyclophosphamide Hexamethylmelamine Adriamycin Cis-platinum	35	49	20	Kane et al 1979
II. HAD Hexamethylmelamine Adriamycin Cis-platinum	22	63	18	Vogl et al 1979
III. HD Hexamethylmelamine Cis-platinum	22	57	20	Davis et al 1980
IV. CHAD Cyclophosphamide Hexamethylmelamine Adriamycin Cis-platinum	20	0	0	Piver et al 1981
V. ACFUCY Actinomycin-D Actinomycin-D 5-Fluorouracil Cyclophosphamide	145	6	<6	Stanhope et al 1977
VI. MECY Methotrexate Cyclophosphamide	47	30	5	Barlow & Piver 1979

combination cyclophosphamide, hexamethylmelamine, adriamycin and cis-platinum (CHAD)* as second-line chemotherapy. In contrast to the results of Kane & Vogl, none of our patients had an objective response (Piver et al 1981).

The reasons for the contrasting results among CHAD, CHAP and HAD are not readily apparent. As seen in Table 7.4, the major differences are the longer periods of infusion of cis-platinum in our study, and our use of pyridoxine to prevent the neurological toxicity of hexamethylmelamine (Johnson et al 1978). Notwithstanding our poor results with CHAD, the reports of hexamethylmelamine plus cis-platinum, CHAP, or HAD, with response rates of 57%, 49% and 63% respectively, and complete clinical responses of 20%, make these regimens the current treatments of

---

* CHAP and CHAD are the same chemotherapeutic regimen, however, some authors refer to the last element, cis-platinum, by the letter D of cis-diaminodichloroplatinum; and others use P to refer to cis-platinum.

Table 7.4 Second-line chemotherapy in ovarian carcinoma (Piver et al 1981)

Days	Drug	CHAD	CHAP	HAD
1	Cis-platinum	1 mg/kg	50 mg/m^2	50 mg/m^2
		5% D/.45NS	5% D/.45NS	5% D/.45NS
		Furosemide	Furosemide	Furosemide
		Mannitol	Mannitol	Mannitol
		6 hours	1 hour	Bolus
	Adriamycin	25 mg/m^2	40 mg/m^2	30 mg/m^2
	Cyclophosphamide	400 mg/m^2	300 mg/m^2	
1–14	Hexamethylmelamine		150 mg/m^2	
8–21		150 mg/m^2		200 mg/m^2
8–21	Pyridoxine	300 mg		
Patients		20	35	22
Response		0%	49%	63%

D = dextrose   NS = normal saline

choice as second-line chemotherapy in advanced ovarian adenocarcinoma.

Third-line chemotherapy

Until recently, there was no effective third-line chemotherapy.
Stanhope et al (1977) reported a response rate of only 4% in 52
patients treated with the combination actinomycin-D, 5-fluorour-
acil and cyclophosphamide (ACFUCY). Because of the effectiveness of cis-platinum as first-line and second-line chemotherapy in
metastatic ovarian adenocarcinomas, we evaluated high-dose cis-
platinum (100 mg/m^2 every three weeks) as third-line chemotherapy (Piver et al 1978). Only one patient (5%) responded.
  Since high-dose cis-platinum was not effective, a study was
initiated to evaluate cis-platinum at a lower dose, (1 mg/kg)
weekly for six weeks, followed by cis-platinum (60 mg/m^2) every
three weeks. We achieved the unusually high partial response rate
of 70% in the first 10 patients treated. This was especially unusual
since all patients had progression of their malignancy after first
and second-line chemotherapy and all had extensive tumour.
Interestingly, of the 10 patients, five had progression of their
malignancy after cis-platinum in the CHAD combination and
three subsequently had a partial response to cis-platinum given on
a weekly basis. Responses lasted from 12 to 33 weeks, and two
patients continued to respond at 20 and 28 weeks respectively, at
the time of the report (Piver et al 1980). The 70% response rate
to weekly cis-platinum compared to the lack of response to high-

dose cis-platinum as third-line chemotherapy is unclear, as is the mechanism of action of response to weekly cis-platinum in patients who had previously failed to respond to cis-platinum given on a monthly basis.

Summary and conclusion

At the present time, the most effective second-line chemotherapeutic regimens against metastatic ovarian adenocarcinoma include the CHAP regimen (cyclophosphamide, hexamethylmelamine, adriamycin and cis-platinum) with an overall response rate of 49%, and a complete response rate of 20%, and the HAD regimen (hexamethylmelamine, adriamycin and cis-platinum) with an overall response rate of 63%, and a complete response rate of 18%. As third-line chemotherapy, the most effective reported regimen to date is the use of weekly cis-platinum as induction therapy for six weeks, followed by either a higher-dose of cis-platinum every three weeks, or the addition of adriamycin and hexamethylmelamine to cis-platinum given every three weeks. More time is required to evaluate the duration of survival after clinical response to second or third-line chemotherapy in metastatic ovarian adenocarcinoma.

REFERENCES

Barlow J J, Piver M S 1979 Second line efficacy of intermediate high dose methotrexate with citrovorum factor rescue cyclophosphamide in ovarian cancer. Gynecologic Oncology 7: 233–238
Bolis G, D'Incalci M, Belloni C, Mangioni C 1979 Hexamethylmelamine in ovarian cancer resistant to cyclophosphamide and adriamycin. Cancer Treatment Reports 63: 1375–1377
Bolis G, D'Incalci M, Gramellini F, Mangioni C 1978 Adriamycin in ovarian cancer patients resistant to cyclophosphamide. European Journal of Cancer 14: 1401–1402
Bonomi P D, Miadineo J, Morrin B, Wilbanks G, Slayton R E 1979 Phase II trial of hexamethylmelamine in ovarian carcinoma resistant to alkylating agents. Cancer Treatment Reports 63: 137–138
Davis T, Vogl S E, Kaplan B H, Tunca J, Arseneau J 1980 Diamminedichloroplatinum (D) and hexamethylmelamine (H) in combination for ovarian cancer (OvCa) after failure of alkylating agent (AA) therapy — a phase I-II pilot trial. Proceedings of American Association of Cancer Research and American Society of Clinical Oncology 20: 428
DePalo G M, De Lena M, Di Re F, Luciani L, Valagussa P, Bonadonna G 1975 Melphalan versus adriamycin in the treatment of advanced carcinoma of the ovary. Surgical Gynecology and Obstetrics 141: 899–902

Second and third-line chemotherapy

Johnson B L, Fisher R I, Bender R A, DeVita V T, Chabner B A, Young R C 1978 Hexamethylmelamine in alkylating agent-resistant ovarian carcinoma. Cancer 42: 2157–2161

Kane R, Harvey H, Andrews T et al 1979 Phase II trial of cyclophosphamide, hexamethylmelamine, adriamycin, and cis-dichlorodiamine platinum (II) combination chemotherapy in advanced ovarian carcinoma. Cancer Treatment Reports 63: 307

Piver M S, Barlow J J, Lele S B, Higby D J 1978 Cis-dichlorodiammine platinum (II) as third line chemotherapy in advanced ovarian adenocarcinoma. Cancer Treatment Reports 62: 559–560

Piver M S, Lele S B, Barlow J J 1980 Weekly cis-diamminoplatinum (II): Active third line chemotherapy in ovarian carcinoma: A preliminary report. Cancer Treatment Reports 64: 71

Piver M S, Lele S B, Barlow J J 1981 Cyclophosphamide, hexamethylmelamine, doxirubicin, and cis-platin (CHAD) as second line chemotherapy for ovarian adenocarcinoma. Cancer Treatment Reports 65: 85

Stanhope C, Smith J P, Rutledge F 1977 Second trial drugs in ovarian cancer. Gynecologic Oncology 5: 52–58

Stehman F, Ballon S, Lagasse L, Chamorro T, Donaldson R, Roberts J, Ford L 1979 Cis-platinum in advanced gynecologic malignancy. Gynecologic Oncology 7: 349–360

Thigpen T, Shingleton H, Homesley H, LaGasse L, Blessing J 1979 Cis-dichlorodiammineplatinum (II) in the treatment of gynecologic malignancies: Phase II trials by the Gynecologic Oncology Group. Cancer Treatment Reports 63: 1549–1555

Vogl S E, Berenzweig M, Kaplan B H, Moukhtar M, Bulkin W 1979 The CHAD and HAD regimens in advanced ovarian cancer: combination chemotherapy including cyclophosphamide, hexamethylmelamine, adriamycin, and cis-dichlorodiammineplatinum (II). Cancer Treatment Reports 63: 311–317

Wiltshaw E, Kroner T 1976 Phase II study of cis-dichlorodiammine platinum (II) (NSC-119875) in advanced adenocarcinoma of the ovary. Cancer Treatment Reports 60: 55–60

8

Second-look laparatomy and second-look laparoscopy in ovarian carcinoma

Introduction

The concept of a second-look laparotomy to evaluate the status of a patient's cancer was introduced by Wangensteen in 1949 for patients with colon carcinoma (Wangensteen et al 1951). This was before the era of effective chemotherapy for malignancies in general and prior to the recent demonstration of highly effective multi-agent chemotherapeutic regimens for ovarian cancer. Since initially there was no effective adjuvant treatment, the purpose of a second-look laparotomy was to determine whether cancer was present, and if so, whether to attempt re-resection. The impetus for a second-look laparotomy in patients with ovarian malignancies occurred in 1961 (Santoro et al 1961) with the development of effective radiation therapy and chemotherapy that could be used to treat any residual ovarian cancer present at the second-look operation. With the development of effective chemotherapy and the complete clinical remissions that resulted, a second-look laparotomy was done before deciding to discontinue chemotherapy in patients with no residual cancer, or to resect residual tumour masses and change the therapy to whole abdominal radiation. This sequential therapy-surgery, followed by chemotherapy, followed by second-look laparotomy, followed by whole abdominal radiation for small residual ovarian malignancy was found to be ineffective in improving survival rates in advanced ovarian carcinoma.

The number of ovarian cancer patients undergoing second-look laparotomies has increased for two reasons. First, a significant incidence of acute nonlymphocytic leukaemia has been reported after prolonged treatment with alkylating agent chemotherapy (Reimer et al 1977). Physicians, therefore, desire to discontinue such therapy at an appropriate time in patients with no evidence of persistent ovarian cancer. Second, the percentage of complete remissions has increased due to the development of effective multiagent chemotherapy for ovarian carcinoma. Physicians are understandably reluctant to stop chemotherapy in patients in complete clinical remission without the benefit of a negative second-look laparotomy, since even one small cluster of tumour cells remaining can result in a recurrence and death.

To evaluate second-look laparotomy as a method to improve the survival rate of women with advanced ovarian adenocarcinoma, we treated patients with sequential therapy consisting of an initial operation, chemotherapy and, in patients in complete clinical remission, a second-look laparotomy, followed by postoperative whole abdominal irradiation. After second-look laparotomy, residual tumour ranged from 0 to less than 2 cm in diameter in all patients (Piver et al 1977). Postoperative whole abdominal irradiation resulted in a five-year survival rate of only 12% in this small series (Piver et al 1977, Piver 1977). In a larger, but similar sequential study, patients found to have residual ovarian cancer at second-look laparotomy were treated with postoperative whole abdominal radiation if the residual cancer was less than 2 cm and with melphalan chemotherapy if more than 2 cm (Smith et al 1976). Even though the melphalan patients had larger residual disease, their 30% five-year survival rate was statistically significantly better ($P<0.01$), compared to the 14% survival rate for those receiving whole abdominal radiation (Table 8.1). The lack of effectiveness of sequential therapy using whole abdominal irradiation has resulted in second-look laparotomy being used primarily for patients in complete clinical remission to confirm that no residual cancer is present, so that chemotherapy can be discontinued.

Table 8.1 Survival by chemotherapy vs. radiation therapy for residual cancer after second-look laparotomy (Smith et al 1976)

Treatment	% 5-year survival
Whole abdominal radiation therapy	14
Phenylalanine mustard (Alkeran, melphalan)	30

Results of second-look laparotomy in ovarian cancer

In 1962, at the M.D. Anderson Hospital and Tumour Institute in Houston, Texas, a prospective programme was initiated to systematically perform a second-look laparotomy on advanced ovarian cancer patients. The results were reported in 1976. The study included 103 women with advanced ovarian cancer who underwent second-look laparotomies after systemic chemotherapy (Smith et al 1976). Early in the study, before guidelines for second-look laparotomy were established, patients underwent the second-look operation when the tumour mass had partially regressed, to attempt a second surgical resection. On the discovery that all such patients had rapid tumour recurrence after second-look laparotomy and resection, the policy was changed and second-look laparotomies were performed only in patients who had complete or near complete clinical response to chemotherapy.

Table 8.2 Survival by number of cycles of chemotherapy prior to second-look laparotomy (Smith et al 1976)

Chemotherapy cycles	% 5-year survival
1–4	9
5–9	32
10 or more	80

This report documents the importance of the timing of second-look laparotomy vis-a-vis chemotherapy. Early in the study, patients who had dramatic responses to chemotherapy, frequently after only several courses of treatment, were subjected to second-look laparotomies at that time. This resulted in early recurrence of the malignancy. As seen in Table 8.2, a significant number of courses of chemotherapy are required to achieve the highest five-year survival rate relative to discontinuation of chemotherapy after a negative second-look laparotomy. Patients receiving one to four courses of chemotherapy had a five-year survival rate of 9%, compared to 32% for five to nine courses and 80% for patients receiving 10 or more courses of monthly chemotherapy. Most importantly, all patients who had a complete response after 12 or more monthly courses of chemotherapy, and who had no residual cancer at second-look laparotomy, were alive at the time of the report.

Second-look laparoscopy prior to proposed second-look laparotomy

If ovarian cancer is present at second-look laparotomy, chemotherapy will be continued, resulting in the need for third- and even fourth-look laparotomies at later dates. Repeated laparotomies must be associated with significant morbidity and even mortality. Therefore, we have evaluated the concept of a second-look laparoscopy prior to second-look laparotomy. If persistent tumour was documented by the second-look laparoscopy, it would spare the patient a formal laparotomy with its attendant morbidity.

Since multiple anaesthesias also have significant morbidity, the plan was to perform a second-look laparoscopy and if no malignancy was present, to perform a second-look laparotomy under the same anaesthetic (Piver et al 1980). Certain patients with no visible tumour at laparoscopy may still have free-floating cancer cells documented cytologically from peritoneal washings. These patients should stay on chemotherapy and do not need a second-look laparotomy. To confirm the presence of these free-floating cells, a special procedure was initiated for the immediate cytological evaluation of peritoneal washings obtained from the pelvis and paracolic spaces during laparoscopy.

At the time of laparoscopy, washings for cytological evaluation were obtained from the pelvis and paracolic spaces by injecting 50 to 100 cc of saline into the pelvis and right and left paracolic spaces. The entire cytological procedure, including preparation and evaluation, takes approximately 30 minutes. All specimens were prepared with a cytocentrifuge and stained with a modified, shortened technique of a classic Papanicolaou smear. Two slides were prepared from each of the three washings (six slides per patient). As seen in Table 8.3 at second-look laparoscopy 36.3% of the patients in complete clinical remission had persistent tum-

Table 8.3 Second-look laparoscopy findings in ovarian adenocarcinoma (Piver et al 1980)

Findings	FIGO stage		Total % (no.)
	IIB	III & IV	
Tumour	0	4	18.1 (4)
Positive cytology	4	3	31.8 (7)
Tumours or positive cytology	4	4	36.3 (8)
Total no. patients	11	11	22

Table 8.4 Incidence of persistent ovarian cancer at second-look laparoscopy (Piver et al 1980)

Authors	No. of patients	Persistent tumour % (no.)
Rosenoff et al	16	31.2 (5)
Piver et al	22	36.3 (8)
Smith et al	24	29.1 (7)
Total	62	32.2 (20)

our. Most importantly, 18% had no visible evidence of ovarian cancer, but had, as their only evidence of persistent tumour, a positive cytological washing.

As seen in Table 8.4, two other studies using second-look laparoscopy in patients in complete clinical remission after chemotherapy for ovarian carcinoma have been reported. Smith et al (1977) reported that 29.1% of their patients had biopsy-proven residual cancer at second-look laparoscopy and were spared second-look laparotomy. However, six of the 24 patients, (25%) with no visible cancer at laparoscopy, had residual malignancy at second-look laparotomy. They did not perform cytological washings at the time of the second-look laparoscopy. Rosenoff et al (1977) performed second-look laparoscopies in patients with advanced ovarian cancer who were in remission for at least one year after initiation of chemotherapy, and 31.2% (5/16) were found to have biopsy-documented residual ovarian cancer at laparoscopy, and thus were continued on chemotherapy. They did not use cytological washings at laparoscopy. Two of four patients who underwent a second-look laparotomy after a negative second-look laparoscopy had microscopic residual cancer present. Therefore, the absence of visible tumour at laparoscopy and the absence of malignant cells on peritoneal washings, allows the physician to proceed with the second-look laparotomy under one anaesthetic. It is axiomatic that if there is no evidence of persistent malignancy at second-look laparoscopy, these patients do require a second-look laparotomy before consideration of discontinuing effective chemotherapy.

Summary and technique

Second-look laparoscopy and laparotomy should be carried out on patients in complete clinical remission after a minimum of 12 monthly courses of chemotherapy. Since approximately one-third of such patients will have persistent tumour demonstrated by the less formidable second-look laparoscopy, this should precede the proposed second-look laparotomy. If no residual ovarian cancer is detected by biopsy or frozen section evaluation of peritoneal washings, the second-look laparotomy should be carried out under the same anaesthetic.

At the time of second-look laparotomy, careful evaluation of the diaphragm, omentum, para-aortic and pelvic lymph nodes should be carried out. In addition, the entire intestine should be carefully evaluated. If the omentum was not resected during the initial procedure, an omentectomy should be performed. Areas where residual ovarian cancer was left in situ at the initial operation should be biopsied even if these areas appear to be normal. Frequently, these peritoneal areas contain small clusters of tumour cells not grossly visible.

REFERENCES

Piver M S 1977 Unpublished data
Piver M S, Barlow J J, Lee F T, Vongtama B 1977 Sequential therapy for advanced ovarian adenocarcinoma: operation, chemotherapy, second-look laparotomy and radiation therapy. American Journal of Obstetrics and Gynecology 122: 355
Piver M S, Lele, S B, Barlow J J, Gamarra M 1980 Second-look laparoscopy prior to proposed second-look laparotomy. Obstetrics and Gynecology 55: 571
Reimer R R, Hoover R, Fraumeni J F et al 1977 Acute leukemia after alkylating-agent therapy of ovarian cancer. New England Journal of Medicine 297: 177
Rosenoff S H, DeVita V T, Hubbard S, Young R C 1977 Peritoneoscopy and staging follow-up of ovarian cancer. Seminars in Oncology 2: 223
Santoro B T, Griffen, W O, Wangensteen O H 1961 The second-look procedure in the management of ovarian malignancies and pseudomixoma peritonei. Surgery 50: 354
Smith W G, Day T G, Smith J P 1977 The use of laparoscopy to determine the results of chemotherapy of ovarian cancer. Journal of Reproductive Medicine 18: 257
Smith J P, Delgado G, Rutledge F 1976 Second-look operation in ovarian carcinoma. Cancer 38: 1438
Wangensteen O H, Lewis F J, Tongen L A 1951 The 'second-look' in cancer surgery. Lancet 71: 303

9

Brenner tumours of the ovary

Introduction

In 1898, McNaughton-Jones first described the ovarian tumours
known today as Brenner tumour, after Brenner reported three
cases in 1907. The World Health Organisation's Classification of
Ovarian Tumours continues to use the name and categorises these
tumours as being either benign, borderline malignant, and malignant.

This classification is used for all common epithelial ovarian
tumours and is based on the premise that Brenner tumours are
derived from Walthard cell islands (rests) from the surface of the
ovarian epithelium. Walthard cell islands, or rests, are embryonic
and have common characteristics with Brenner cells, including
longitudinal grooving of the nuclei, cystic formation and mucin
secretion. Comparing the light and ultrastructural features of the
two, Bransilver et al (1974) reported that a close resemblance
exists between Walthard rests and Brenner tumours, and that they
are derived from the celomic epithelium of the ovary. It is currently accepted, therefore, that the histogenesis of Brenner
tumours is from the surface epithelium of the ovary.

Brenner tumours account for 2% of all ovarian tumours. From
a clinical standpoint, it is significant that 99% are benign. The
majority of these tumours are approximately 5 cm in diameter but
they have been described as large as 25 to 30 cm in diameter.
Brenner tumour patients are usually asymptomatic and 95% of
these tumours are found incidentally at surgery for unrelated problems.

Rarely, patients with Brenner tumours present with abdominal
pain and swelling secondary to benign ascites and hydrothorax

(Meigs syndrome). Abnormal uterine bleeding has been the presenting symptom in 10 to 15% of these patients. Similarly, 15% have endometrial hyperplasia and only rarely have endometrial carcinoma. Despite the incidence of abnormal uterine bleeding, endometrial hyperplasia and occasional endometrial carcinoma, there is no direct hormonal evidence that Brenner tumours are oestrogen producing.

Brenner tumours consist of multiple epithelial solid nests within a fibrous stroma similar to transitional cell epithelium and have the appearance of a low-grade papillary transitional cell carcinoma of the bladder. Rarely, the fibrous stroma also contains Leydig cell hyperplasia or stromal leutinisation. A diagnosis of malignant Brenner tumour is made when a transition between benign and malignant elements is present.

A major complication in the care of Brenner tumour patients is that approximately 15–30% of these tumours are associated with another tumour in the opposite ovary. Most commonly, these tumours are either a mucinous or a serous cystadenoma, and less commonly, they are either a mature cystic teratoma or a cystadenocarcinoma. Waxman (1979) reviewed 460 Brenner tumour cases and found that 66 (14.3%) were associated with a mucinous cystadenoma, or less commonly, a cystadenocarcinoma or serous cystadenoma. More significantly, 23% of these patients had an associated gynaecological or systemic malignancy. Similarly, Silverberg (1971) found a 22% (12) incidence of other malignancies in 54 Brenner tumour patients. Balasa et al (1977) reviewed 302 Brenner tumour cases and found that there were concomitant neoplasms in 100 (30%), with a serous or a mucinous cystadenoma the most common (58%). The significant association with surface derived neoplasms further stresses the theory that Brenner tumours originate from the surface of the ovarian epithelium. However, the association of Brenner tumours with other malignancies probably reflects the fact that Brenner tumours are found incidentally at surgery for unrelated problems, rather than that there is a causal relationship to the other malignancies.

Borderline or proliferative Brenner tumours

Borderline malignant or 'proliferative' Brenner tumours are rare and account for less than 1% of all Brenner tumours. In 1971, Roth & Sternberg were among the first to suggest a separate category of 'proliferative' Brenner tumours. This intermediate category between benign and malignant Brenner tumours is characterised by a papillary intracystic pattern with rare mitosis and minimal cellular atypia but with no invasion of the ovarian stroma. Hallgrimsson & Scully (1972) suggested the term Brenner tumour of 'borderline malignancy' rather than 'proliferative' Brenner tumour to comply with the International Federation of Gynecology Obstetrics (FIGO) classification of other ovarian tumours derived from ovarian surface epithelium.

These authors have all reported that Brenner tumours of borderline malignancy have been unilateral, mostly cystic and measuring approximately 8 to 10 cm in diameter. Since the original three cases reported by Roth & Sternberg, Balasa et al were able to collect another 15 cases of Brenner tumours of borderline malignancy. The patients ranged in age from 30 to 87, with a median age of 45 to 50. Symptoms included vaginal bleeding, increased abdominal girth and on a rare occasion, Meigs syndrome.

Originally, the Brenner tumours of borderline malignancy were considered to be benign because of the lack of significant epithelial anaplasia, invasion, metastasis and the lack of documented recurrences. Of the seven borderline malignant tumours reported by Miles & Norris (1972), all were FIGO stage IA at the initial operation and all patients were alive and well 2.5 to 13.5 years after treatment by surgery alone. Notwithstanding the benign nature of the cases reported by Miles & Norris and others, Pratt-Thomas and coauthors (1976) recently reported a patient with a stage IA Brenner tumour of borderline malignancy diagnosed by light and electron microscopy, and treated by surgery and strip irradiation to the entire abdomen, who developed extensive liver metastasis six years after completing this therapy.

Malignant Brenner tumours

Prior to 1945, all Brenner tumours were considered to be benign. In 1945, von Numers reported the first two cases of malignant Brenner tumours, and in 1971, Roth & Sternberg reported the first cases of Brenner tumours of borderline malignancy. Recently, Pratt-Thomas and coauthors (1976) reviewed all of the reported cases of malignant Brenner tumours and felt that only 48 filled the criteria of malignant Brenner tumours. Most reports of malignant Brenner tumours were individual case reports until the eight cases reported by Hallgrimsson & Scully (1972) and the seven cases by Miles & Norris, (1972). The median age of patients with malignant Brenner tumours was approximately 60 to 68, which is significantly higher than the median of patients with Brenner tumours of borderline malignancy (50).

Of the seven cases reported by Miles & Norris, three patients died in less than two years. Follow-up of the eight cases of Hallgrimsson & Scully revealed that two of three patients died at 20 and 41 months, respectively, when there was malignant Brenner tumour without associated concomitant benign elements present within the ovary. In contrast, the other five patients with associated benign elements were without evidence of recurrence from six months to 12 years after surgery. Most likely, this contrast in survival was coincidental rather than a biological effect of the benign elements on the behaviour of malignant Brenner tumours. Of the malignant Brenner tumours reported by Miles & Norris, six patients had FIGO stage I disease and two died at one and two years following treatment by surgery and surgery alone, and two patients were alive without evidence of recurrence at five months and 3.5 years, following treatment by surgery alone. One patient with stage III malignant Brenner tumour treated by surgery alone died at three months.

Radiation and chemotherapy

There is very little information on the use of postoperative radiation therapy and there are no data on the use of chemotherapy in patients with borderline malignant or malignant Brenner tumours. Anecdotally, Shay & Janovski (1963) reported a patient with Brenner tumour treated by 4000 rads to the pelvis but no follow-up was recorded. Hull & Campbell (1973) reported a patient treated with radiation therapy for recurrent malignant Brenner tumour who did not respond. Rawson & Helman (1955) reported a patient treated with 1500 rads, who did not respond. The patient treated by Balasa et al (1977), received 4000 rad to the pelvis but had recurrence in the pelvis, abdomen, liver and pleura.

Finally, Pratt-Thomas et al (1976) reported a patient with stage I malignant Brenner tumour who had associated non-malignant ascites and pleural effusion treated by strip irradiation to the whole abdomen. The patient was well one year after treatment and the symptoms of Meigs syndrome regressed.

Treatment and conclusion

It is clear that these individual reports on the use of postoperative radiation in patients with malignant Brenner tumours do not allow for an establishment of guidelines. However, since Brenner tumours are considered to be common epithelial tumours of the ovary, the principles established for other common epithelial tumours should be applied to malignant Brenner tumours. Finally, since 99% of Brenner tumours are benign, they should be treated conservatively by unilateral salpingo-oophorectomy in the young patient. However, it is significant that 15 to 30% of the patients with Brenner tumours have a concomitant tumour in the opposite ovary. Therefore, in such instances a wedge biopsy of the ovary should be considered. Patients with borderline malignant Brenner tumours or malignant Brenner tumours should be treated stage for stage as patients with borderline or malignant epithelial tumours of the ovary.

REFERENCES

Balasa R W, Adcock L L, Prem K A, Dehner L P 1977 The Brenner tumour. A clinicopathologic review. Obstetrics and Gynecology 50: 120

Bransilver B R, Ferenczy A, Richart R M 1974 Brenner tumours and Walthard cell nests. Archives of Pathology 98: 76

Brenner F 1907 Das Oophorama follicular. Frankfurter Zeitschrift für Pathologie 1: 150

Hallgrimsson J, Scully R E 1972 Borderline and malignant Brenner tumours of the ovary. Acta pathologica et microbiologica scandinavica section A 80: 233: 56

Hull G R, Campbell G R 1973 The malignant Brenner tumour. Obstetrics and Gynecology 42: 527

McNaughton-Jones H 1898 Uterine fibroids with anomalous ovarian tumours. Transactions of the London Obstetrics Society 40: 154

Miles P A, Norris H J 1972 Proliferative and malignant Brenner tumours of the ovary. Cancer 30: 174

von Numers C 1945 A contribution to the case knowledge and histology of the Brenner tumour. Do malignant forms of the Brenner tumour also occur? Acta obstetrica et gynecologica scandinavica 25: Suppl. 2: 114

Pratt-Thomas H R, Kreutner A, Underwood P B, Dowdeswell R H 1976 Proliferative and malignant Brenner tumours of the ovary. Gynecologic Oncology 4: 176

Rawson A J, Helman M R 1955 Malignant Brenner tumour, Report of a case. American Journal of Obstetrics and Gynecology 69: 429

Roth L M, Sternberg W H 1971 Proliferative Brenner tumour. Cancer 27: 687

Shay M D, Janovski N A 1963 Malignant Brenner tumour associated with endometrial adenocarcinoma. Obstetrics and Gynecology 22: 246

Silverberg S G 1971 Brenner tumour of the ovary. A clinicopathologic study of 60 tumours in 54 women. Cancer 28: 588

Waxman M 1979 Pure and mixed Brenner tumours of the ovary. Cancer 43: 1830

10

Immature ovarian teratomas

Introduction

Immature teratoma is a germ cell tumour composed of tissue from all three germ layers (endoderm, ectoderm and mesoderm), with at least one cell type immature or incomplete in its differentiation. Prior to the 1973 World Health Organisation's Classification of ovarian tumours, immature teratomas were known as either solid, malignant, embryonal teratoma, teratocarcinoma or teratoblastoma. Since immature teratomas are at least partially cystic, the term solid was inappropriate. Although the malignant areas are embryonal, the term embryonal teratoma was often confused with embryonal carcinoma. However, since it is the immaturity of the tissue that determines its ability to metastasise, the World Health Organisation formulated the term immature teratoma.

Immature teratomas occur primarily in the young, whose future fertility is important when deciding therapy. They are the third most frequent germ cell tumour of the ovary, ranking after dysgerminoma and endodermal sinus tumour. Immature teratomas account for approximately 15% of all germ-cell tumours and 1% of all teratomas. Histologically, immature neural tissues are the most common immature tissues present.

Two important reports have improved our understanding of immature teratomas and have resulted in significant improvement in survival of children with this malignancy. The findings indicate that survival and treatment of these tumours are related to the grade of the tumour, i.e., the amount of immature tissue present, and that combination chemotherapy can result in a long-term survival and actual cure.

Grade and survival

In 1960, Thurnbeck & Scully reported a grading system for ovarian teratomas based on the amount of immature tissue within the tumour. Grade 0 teratomas consist of only mature tissues and have no known malignant potential. Grade 1 teratomas contain small amounts of immature tissue, frequently immature neural epithelium, or cartilage with rare mitosis; grade 2 teratomas contain a moderate amount of immature elements; whereas grade 3 tumours contain large amounts of immature or embryonal tissues with numerous mitosis (Table 10.1).

Table 10.1 Grading of ovarian teratomas (Thurnbeck and Scully 1960)

Grade 0	All tissues mature: no mitotic activity
Grade 1	Minor foci of embryonal tissue: rare mitosis
Grade 2	Moderate quantities of embryonal tissue: moderate mitotic activity
Grade 3	Large quantities of embryonal tissue

The lack of malignant potential is demonstrated in the report of 15 grade 0 ovarian teratomas by Woodruff and coauthors (1968). Fourteen patients were alive and well and one was lost to follow-up. None had recurrent disease. Teratomas composed entirely of grade 0 elements, therefore, are almost without exception, benign tumours that are associated with long-term survival and require only surgical removal. However, patients with grade 1, 2 or 3 tumours frequently do not do well when treated by surgery alone. This was especially true before the recent development of effective combination chemotherapy and was demonstrated in an earlier report of 19 patients with malignant ovarian teratomas, the majority of whom were dead in one year (Malkasian et al 1965). Only two patients survived.

Norris and coauthors (1976), using a modified Thurnbeck-Scully grading system with their addition of quantification of the amount of neural tissue within the tumour, demonstrated clearly the relationship between the grade of the immature teratoma and ultimate survival. Of their 40 patients with stage I immature teratoma, 85% (34) were treated by unilateral salpingo-oophorectomy. Survival without evidence of disease for stage I, grade 1 was 100%, for grade 2 55%, and for grade 3 33% (Table 10.2). Of the patients with metastasis (stages II and III), and in whom tissue was available for grading the metastasis, all of the patients with grade 0 tumours were alive without evidence of tumour more than seven

Table 10.2 Stage I immature ovarian teratomas: survival vs. grade (Norris et al 1976)

Grade	Patients	Survival NED* (%)
1	14	100
2	20	55
3	6	33

* NED = no evidence of disease

years, in contrast to less than 50% of the grade 1 and 2 tumours, and none of the patients with grade 3 tumours. Since the grade of the tumour is most important in gauging prognosis and deciding on therapy, one block of tumour should be examined for every centimeter of tumour. If metastasis is present, it is imperative to biopsy and grade multiple implants.

Combination chemotherapy and survival

We have treated five children, ages 11 to 17, who originally had stage IA immature teratoma of the ovary. None of the five children received adjuvant therapy after the initial surgery and all five developed abdominal recurrences within 10 months of initial surgery (Piver & Lurain 1979). These children were subsequently treated with combination chemotherapy consisting primarily of vincristine, actinomycin-D and cyclophosphamide (VAC). Two of our patients are surviving without evidence of tumour 5 and 10 years respectively, after combination chemotherapy for stage III,

Table 10.3 Stage IA ovarian immature teratoma in 11–17 years old patients (Piver & Lurain 1979)

Stage	Primary adjunctive treatment	Recurrence (months)	Number of patients-treatment of recurrence	Status (months)
IA	none	2	VAC	NED (120)
IA	none	6	VAC	NED (60)
IA	none	10	1. VAC	...
			2. Isophosphamide	DOD (78)
IA	none	2	VAC	DOD (7)
IA	none	9	VAC	DOD (11)

VAC = vincristine, actinomycin-D, cyclophosphamide
NED = no evidence of disease
DOD = dead of disease

grade 2 or 3 immature teratoma of the ovary (Table 10.3). In both cases, the immature tissues (grade 2 and 3) matured to grade 0 peritoneal implants after combination chemotherapy (Piver et al 1976).

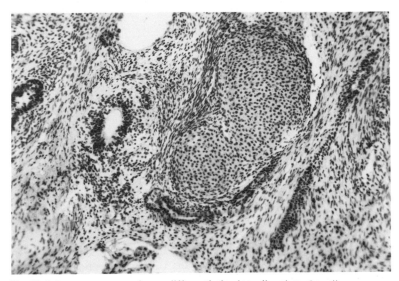

Fig. 10.1 Immature mesenchyme differentiating into direction of cartilage (× 160). Reprinted by permission of Cancer

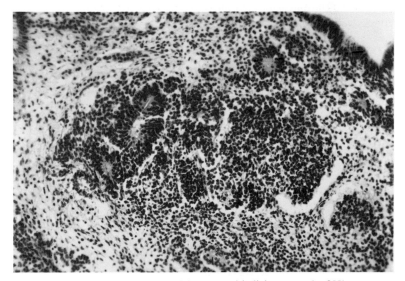

Fig. 10.2 Immature neural tissue with neuroepithelial rosettes (× 200). Reprinted by permission of Cancer

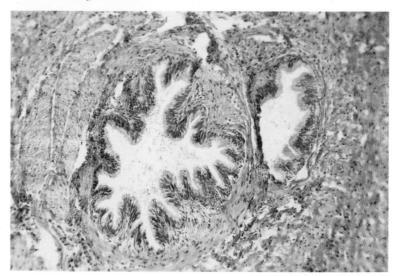

Fig. 10.3 Glands lined by respiratory epithelium and surrounded by mature fibromuscular tissue (× 160). Reprinted by permission of Cancer

Figures 10.1 and 10.2 demonstrate the immature cartilage and neural tissues prior to the initiation of VAC chemotherapy. Figure 10.3 demonstrates that only grade 0 tissue is present at the second-look laparotomy after successful combination chemotherapy. Currently, the patient is off chemotherapy for seven years and is surviving without recurrent immature teratoma of the ovary. This conversion of immature metastatic teratoma to mature teratoma by VAC chemotherapy has been reported by other investigators (DiSaia et al 1977, Cangir et al 1978). Cangir and coauthors reported on the use of VAC chemotherapy in eight children, 16 years old and younger, who had immature ovarian teratoma. All eight were alive without tumour at 24 to 80 months after treat-

Table 10.4 VAC chemotherapy and second-look operative findings (Cangir et al 1978)

Stage	Second-look operation	Survival (months)
I	Grade 0 glial implants	52+
I	No tumour	32+
I	No tumour	35+
I	Grade 0 glial implants	24+
I	No tumour	55+
II	Grade 0 glial implants	80+
III	Grade 0 glial implants	78+
III	Grade 0 ganglioneuroma	25+

ment. At second-look laparotomy, six of the eight patients had persistent grade 0 implants, including all three patients with stage II and III disease (Table 10.4).

Another report of the efficacy of VAC chemotherapy was that of Curry and coauthors (1978) who reported 10 patients with stage II, III and IV immature teratoma. Seven of the 10 are alive without evidence of cancer from 16 to 68 months after treatment. This is in contrast to the 100% mortality in their earlier study of 13 patients with immature teratoma who were treated prior to VAC (Table 10.5).

Table 10.5 Survival after VAC chemotherapy (Curry et al 1978)

Stage	Survival NED (months)	Alive* or Dead with Cancer (months)
IIA	43	
III	16, 20, 40, 43, 48	3, 26
IV	68	38*

It is clear, therefore, that VAC chemotherapy will result in long-term survival and cure of young patients with metastatic immature teratoma of the ovary. Moreover, its use as adjuvant therapy for stage I, grade 1, 2 or 3 immature teratoma should prevent recurrences in most young patients with this disease. Since immature teratomas are rarely bilateral and occur most frequently in the young, surgical treatment by unilateral salpingo-oophorectomy, followed by adjuvant VAC chemotherapy allows for preservation of future fertility (Table 10.6).

Table 10.6 VAC chemotherapy

Drug	VAC	Modified VAC
Vincristine	1.5 mg/m^2 weekly × 12 (Not to exceed 2 mg)	Same
Actinomycin-D	0.5 mg i.v. daily × 5 every 4 weeks for 1–2 years	0.009 mg/kg i.v. daily × 5 every 6 weeks
Cyclophosphamide	7 mg/kg i.v. daily × 5 every 4 weeks for 1–2 years	10 mg/kg i.v. daily × 5 every 6 weeks

REFERENCES

Cangir A, Smith J, Van Eys J 1978 Improved prognosis in children with ovarian cancers following modified VAC (Vincristine sulfate, Dactinomycin, and Cyclophosphamide) chemotherapy. Cancer 42: 1234

Curry S L, Smith J P, Gallagher H W 1978 Malignant teratoma of the ovary: prognostic factors and treatment. American Journal of Obstetrics and Gynecology 131: 845

DiSaia P H, Saltz A, Kagan A R, Morrow C P 1977 Chemotherapeutic retroconversion of immature teratoma of the ovary. Obstetrics and Gynecology 49: 346

Malkasian G D, Symmonds R E, Dockerty M B 1965 Malignant ovarian teratomas — report of 31 cases. Obstetrics and Gynecology 25: 810–814

Norris H J, Zirkin H J, Benson W L 1976 Immature (malignant) teratoma of the ovary. Cancer 37: 2359

Piver M S, Lurain J 1979 Childhood ovarian cancers — new advances in treatment. New York State Journal of Medicine 79: 1196

Piver M S, Sinks, L, Barlow J J, Tsukada Y 1976 Five-year remissions of metastatic solid teratoma of the ovary. Cancer 38: 987

Thurnbeck W M, Scully R E 1960 Solid teratoma of the ovary — a clinicopathological analysis of 9 cases. Cancer 13: 804

Woodruff J D, Protos P, Peterson W F 1968 Ovarian teratomas. Relationship of histologic and ontogenic factors for prognosis. American Journal of Obstetrics and Gynecology 102: 702

11

Endodermal sinus tumour and embryonal carcinoma of the ovary

Introduction

Endodermal sinus tumour is the second most common malignant germ-cell tumour of the ovary. Confusion still exists regarding the management of the tumour, because of the numerous names applied to it in the past. It has been classified as embryonal carcinoma, extraembryonal teratoma, yolk sac tumour, immature mesonephroma, mesoblastoma vittelinum, extraembryonal mesoblastoma and Teilum tumour.

Historically, three important events have helped to clarify our understanding of this tumour; Schiller (1939) first described the tumour; Teilum (1959) classified it as endodermal sinus tumour of the ovary and Kurman & Norris (1976a,b) described and separated the less common embryonal carcinoma from endodermal sinus tumour.

In 1939, Schiller described two ovarian tumours under the name mesonephroma ovarii. One of these tumours is now referred to as endodermal sinus tumour but also includes examples of embryonal carcinoma. The second was also originally named mesonephroma but was later discovered not to be a germ-cell tumour, but rather a clear-cell ovarian adenocarcinoma.

In 1959, Gunnar Teilum coined the term endodermal sinus tumour in his classification of germ-cell tumours. He separated germ-cell tumours into those arising from extraembryonic structures (endodermal sinus tumour and choriocarcinoma), such as the yolk sac and allantois, and those arising from the embryo (teratomas). He named the tumour endodermal sinus tumour because it resembles the endodermal sinus of the rodent placenta which had been previously described by Duval. Seen histologically, the endodermal sinus is referred to as the Schiller Duval body, and consists of layers of primitive germ cells with a central capillary. This pattern occurs in 75% of endodermal sinus tumours, but is not often seen in the less common polyvesicular vitteline pattern, which consists of primitive cells surrounding a cystic space or, the least common, solid pattern of endodermal sinus tumours.

In 1976, Kurman & Norris described 15 cases of the ovarian germ-cell tumour now referred to as embryonal carcinoma, separating them histologically, immunohistochemically and clinically from the more common endodermal sinus tumour of the ovary. Embryonal carcinoma of the ovary resembles the embryonal carcinoma of the adult testes, whereas the endodermal sinus tumour has the appearance of the endodermal sinus tumour of the infantile testes. There are also differences in age, incidence, hormonal activity, survival and possibly, in therapeutic management between the two. The Schiller-Duval bodies of the endodermal sinus tumour are not seen in embryonal carcinoma, which is composed primarily of solid sheets of germ cells. Using special histochemical techniques (immunoperoxidase), Kurman & Norris were able to demonstrate alpha-fetoprotein (AFP) and beta-subunit human chorionic gonadotrophin (HCG) in the tumour tissue of embryonal carcinomas, but only AFP in the endodermal sinus tumours. Both groups of tumours, however, were associated with elevated serum levels of AFP. Because of the HCG activity in embryonal carcinoma, patients frequently have hormonal manifestations as well as positive pregnancy tests. All of the patients with embryonal carcinoma reported by Kurman & Norris had positive pregnancy tests and histochemical evidence of HCG in the tumour tissue.

In addition to separating embryonal carcinoma from endodermal sinus tumour, the authors believe that embryonal carcinoma, in spite of the tissue and clinical manifestations of HCG, can be distinguished from ovarian choriocarcinoma. Histologically, embryonal carcinoma lacks the excessive amount of haemorrhage and the syncytiotrophoblasts associated with ovarian choriocarcinoma. Syncytiotrophoblasts were not seen in any of the 15 embryonal carcinomas described. However, scattered throughout the tumours were multinucleated giant cells which did resemble syncytial cells. Endodermal sinus tumours represented 22% and embryonal carcinomas 5% of the ovarian malignant germ-cell tumours in this Armed Forces Institute of Pathology study by Kurman & Norris. Endodermal sinus tumour ranked second in frequency to dysgerminoma and was more frequent than immature teratoma.

Age, symptoms and stage at presentation

In a report by Shrikhande & Sirsat (1975) of 27 endodermal sinus tumour cases, 59% occurred in the second decade, the youngest was 11 months and the oldest 31 years. In the Kurman & Norris study (1976b), the endodermal sinus tumour patients ranged in age from 14 months to 45 years, with a median age of 19. Very few patients were over 40 years of age. In contrast, the 15 patients with embryonal carcinoma reported by Kurman & Norris (1976a) ranged from 4 to 28 years, with a median age of 15. In the literature review of 150 cases of pure endodermal sinus tumour by Gallion et al (1979) the age of the patients ranged from 2 to 45 years, with a median age of 18. Two-thirds of the cases occurred in patients less than 20 years of age, (Table 11.1).

Table 11.1 Comparison of characteristics between endodermal sinus tumour and embryonal carcinoma (Kurman & Norris 1976a & 1976b)

Characteristics	Endodermal sinus tumour	Embryonal carcinoma
Median age	19 years	15 years
% Malignant ovarian germ Cell tumours	22%	5%
Precocious puberty	–	+
Abnormal menstruation	–	+
Pregnancy test	–	+
Serum AFP	+	+
Tumour AFP	+	+
Tumour HCG	–	+

Kurman & Norris reported that 60% of their embryonal carcinoma patients had hormonal manifestations consisting of precocious puberty in the premenarchial girls, abnormal vaginal bleeding in postmenarchial women, and positive pregnancy tests. In contrast, patients with endodermal sinus tumour have negative pregnancy tests. The previous reports of possible hormonal activity in endodermal sinus tumours, probably represented ovarian choriocarcinoma or embryonal carcinoma (Table 11.1).

Because these tumours grow rapidly, symptoms are usually of short duration (2–4 weeks). Most of the children first experience abdominal pain. Even though they are rapidly expanding tumours, 75% of the Kurman & Norris series were stage IA at initial diagnosis. Unless there is peritoneal metastasis present initially, bilateral ovarian involvement by endodermal sinus tumour or embryonal carcinoma is very rare. However, of the 71 endodermal sinus tumours described by Kurman & Norris, five did have a benign cystic teratoma in the opposite ovary and 10 had an ipsilateral benign teratoma. In the literature review of Gallion, 60% of the endodermal sinus tumours were confined to the ovary at initial diagnosis.

Survival

Until the recent discovery of the efficacy of adjuvant combination chemotherapy in the treatment of endodermal sinus tumours and embryonal carcinomas, the prognosis was extremely poor even when the tumour was clinically confined to the ovary at initial diagnosis. This is documented in the following five series, in which most of the patients were treated prior to the era of effective combination chemotherapy. Jimerson & Woodruff (1977) reported a two-year survival rate of 8.8% (3/34), with the three survivors all having stage I tumours. Kurman & Norris (1976b) reported an actuarial survival rate of 13% at three years for patients with endodermal sinus tumour, and eight of their nine survivors had stage I tumours. They reported that 84% of their stage I endodermal sinus tumour patients died of metastasis. In contrast, the actuarial survival rate for their patients with embryonal carcinoma was 39%, and 50% for those with stage I tumours (Kurman & Norris 1976a). Shrikhande & Sirsat (1975) reported on 14 patients available for follow-up. Seven died within six months of diagnosis, two died within one year of diagnosis, and four developed metastasis or recurrence within a short period of time. Only one patient was alive 1.5 years after surgery. In 1975, Forney et al reviewed 102 cases of endodermal sinus tumour of the ovary and all but 10 were dead within two years of diagnosis, and all 10 survivors had stage IA disease. Seven of the survivors had only a small focus of endodermal sinus tumour associated with a well encapsulated dysgerminoma. In the review by Gallion et al (1979), the two-year survival rate for stage I pure endodermal sinus tumours was only 27%, of whom 15% died within a year of diagnosis. The 27% survival rate for stage I tumours was not significantly different from the 33% survival rate for stage II, and the 21% survival rate for stage III tumours. Of those treated by unilateral salpingo-oophorectomy, the two-year survival rate was 16%, and was no better than those treated by hysterectomy and bilateral salpingo-oophorectomy (13%). Only 3% (1/40) treated by surgery and pelvic or abdominal radiation survived two years after treatment. This is in contrast to the over 65% of patients alive two or more years after combination chemotherapy using vincristine, actinomycin-D and cyclophosphamide (VAC).

VAC chemotherapy and surgical therapy

Vincristine, actinomycin-D and cyclophosphamide (VAC) chemotherapy was used initially in endomdermal sinus tumours and embryonal carcinoma because these chemical agents were active, both as single agents and in combination, in treating other embryonal tumours such as embryonal rhabdomyosarcoma, Ewing sarcoma, Wilms tumour, neuroblastoma, and testicular germ-cell tumours (Table 11.2).

Table 11.2 VAC chemotherapy

Drug	VAC	Modified VAC
Vincristine	1.5 mg/m^2 Weekly × 12 (Not to exceed 2 mg)	Same
Actinomycin-D	0.5 mg i.v. Daily × 5 every 4 Weeks for 1–2 years	0.009 mg/kg i.v. Daily × 5 every 6 weeks
Cyclophosphamide	7 mg/kg i.v. Daily × 5 every 4 weeks for 1–2 years	10 mg/kg i.v. Daily × 5 every 6 weeks

In the report of Smith & Rutledge (1975), the efficacy of VAC chemotherapy was demonstrated with apparent cures of 15 of 20 patients treated. Seven of seven stage I patients, two of two stage II patients, five of eight stage III patients, and one of three stage IV patients were alive without evidence of disease at 3 to 78 months after VAC chemotherapy. This is in contrast to virtually no survivors following treatment with actinomycin-D, 5-fluorouracil and cyclophosphamide (ACFUCY); actinomycin-D, methotrexate, and chlorambucil; radiation therapy; or single-agent chemotherapy. However, follow-up was variable and ranged from 3 to 78 months. Moreover, these authors used the term embryonal carcinoma to include both endodermal sinus tumour and embryonal carcinoma so that the specific effectiveness of VAC on either tumour is not evident (Table 11.3).

Table 11.3 Endodermal sinus tumour of the ovary: survival. M.D. Anderson Hospital and Tumor Institute 1947–1974 (Smith & Rutledge 1975)

| Treatment | Stage | | | | |
	I	II	III	IV	Total
Radiation therapy	1/3	0	0/9	0/2	1/14
VAC	7/7	2/2	5/8	1/3	15/20
ACFUCY	0	0/1	1/4	0/3	1/8
ACT-D, MTX, CHLOR.	0	0	0/1	0/1	0/2
Alkylating agent	0	0	0/3	0	0/3
None	1/1	0	0	0	1/1
Total	9/11	2/3	6/25	1/9	18/48

We have used VAC chemotherapy in endodermal sinus tumour of the ovary in nine children 4 to 18 years of age, but could only achieve long-term survival in those children who had no residual endodermal sinus tumour prior to initiation of VAC chemotherapy; i.e., two stage IA and one stage IIB patients (Table 11.4). The remaining six patients with stages IIB–IV did not respond to VAC chemotherapy and all were dead within 4 to 24 months (Piver & Lurain 1979).

Table 11.4 VAC chemotherapy: survival (Piver & Lurain 1979)

Stage	Response (months)	Status (months)
IA	–	NED (75)
IA	–	NED (46)
IIB	CR (23)	NED (23)
IIB	P	DOD (4)
IIB	S (3)	DOD (6)
III	S (13)	DOD (13)
III	S (17)	DOD (24)
III	P	DOD (7)
IV	P	DOD (10)

NED = no evidence of disease   DOD = dead of disease   CR = complete response   P = Progressive   S = Stationary disease

In the literature review by Gallion et al (1979), the highest survival rate resulted from VAC chemotherapy, which was significantly ($P<0.001$) more effective than any other drug regimen, resulting in remissions lasting over two years. Two-thirds of the patients were alive two or more years following initial VAC chemotherapy treatment.

The lack of possible efficacy of VAC chemotherapy was pointed out in the Slayton study of 11 stage IA patients with endodermal sinus tumours treated with VAC chemotherapy. Five patients,

45%, had progression of their malignancy within 12 months of treatment, and six patients were clinically free of disease, with a median follow-up of 19 months (Slayton et al 1978). It may be that as longer follow-up of these patients is obtained, more patients with the earliest stage IA endodermal sinus tumours will develop recurrences, negating the value of adjuvant VAC chemotherapy.

Vinblastine, bleomycin and cis-platinum (VBP) combination chemotherapy

Although VAC chemotherapy appears to have improved the prognosis for some patients with endodermal sinus tumour or embryonal carcinoma, the important study by Einhorn & Donahue (1977), using vinblastine, bleomycin and cis-platinum (VBP) in disseminated non-seminomatous germ-cell testicular carcinomas, may indeed significantly improve the prognosis for young girls with ovarian endodermal sinus tumours or embryonal carcinomas. They treated 47 patients with VBP, and 98% (46) responded, including 72% complete remissions (34) and 26% partial remissions (12). Moreover, five of these 12 patients with partial responses achieved complete remission after subsequent surgery. Of these germ-cell tumours of the testes, two were pure endodermal sinus tumours, and both patients had complete remissions. This outstanding success of VBP in treating testicular carcinomas led to its use in ovarian germ-cell tumours (Table 11.5).

Table 11.5 Vinblastine, bleomycin, cis-platinum treatment programme

---

Days 1, 2, 3, 4, 5:
    1) Hydration & diuresis prior to cis-platinum:
       A) 1000 cc 5% d/w + 36 g Mannitol over 6 h
       B) 40 mg Lasix 1 hour prior to cis-platinum
Day 1: Vinblastine 0.15 mg/kg i.v. infusion for 15 min
       Cis-Platinum 20 mg/m^2 i.v. infusion for 15 min
Day 2: Vinblastine 0.15 mg/kg i.v. infusion for 15 min
       Cis-Platinum 20 mg/m^2 i.v. infusion for 15 min
       Bleomycin 30 mg i.v.
Days 3, 4, 5: Cis-Platinum 20 mg/m^2 i.v. infusion for 15 min
Days 9 and 16: Bleomycin 30 mg* i.v.
Day 22: Repeat cycle

---

* Maximum total dose of 360 mg

In a report by Julian and coauthors (1980), two patients with large residual disease (10 cm and 9 cm tumours, respectively) were treated with VBP, and had a complete response as documented by second-look laparotomy and normalisation of alpha-fetoprotein levels. Both patients are off chemotherapy without evidence of recurrent tumour. In a recent report of the efficacy of VBP in germ-cell tumours of the ovary in advanced disease (stages I, II, IV or recurrent), Williams and coauthors (1981) reported that 10 of 11 patients responded, including six complete responses.

Serum alpha-fetoprotein and response to therapy

Serum alpha-fetoprotein (AFP) levels are elevated in patients with endodermal sinus tumour or embryonal carcinoma. Moreover, Talermann et al (1978) noted elevated AFP levels even prior to clinical evidence of tumour. AFP levels decrease to normal after surgical removal of an endodermal sinus tumour or embryonal carcinoma. However, Sell and coauthors (1976) did report one patient who died with widespread endodermal sinus tumour who had only minimal AFP elevation.

Surgery for endodermal sinus tumours

An important part of understanding the management of children with endodermal sinus tumours came from Forney (1978) who reported the first case of successful pregnancy after unilateral salpingo-oophorectomy and combination chemotherapy for treatment of endodermal sinus tumour of the ovary. At the time of his report, the patient was without evidence of tumours for 2.5 years after the original surgery. Since these tumours are almost never bilateral, and since there is now effective adjuvant chemotherapy, future fertility can by preserved by performing a unilateral salpingo-oophorectomy only.

Surgery for embryonal carcinoma

The surgical management of stage IA embryonal carcinoma remains unilateral salpingo-oophorectomy. In the report of Kurman & Norris (1976a), two-thirds of the embryonal carcinomas in their series were stage I and none were bilateral. However, the normal appearing ovary should be biopsied because a small portion of embryonal carcinomas may have subclinical dysgerminomas admixed with embryonal carcinoma, which may not be detected on frozen section diagnosis. Since dysgerminomas have a high frequency of bilaterality, an unrecognised dysgerminoma at the time of initial surgery may result in missing a dysgerminoma in the opposite ovary.

Summary and conclusion

Although the prognosis for young girls with endodermal sinus tumour or embryonal carcinoma was extremely poor, the recent discovery of effective chemotherapy consisting of vincristine, actinomycin-D and cyclophosphamide (VAC), or vinblastine, bleomycin and cis-platinum (VBP), has resulted in a dramatic reversal. Moreover, since these tumours are rarely bilateral, fertility can be preserved in stage I tumours by performing an unilateral salpingo-oophorectomy, followed by combination chemotherapy with VAC or VBP. These tumours can be monitored by serum alpha-fetoprotein (AFP) levels, and chemotherapy can be discontinued after normalisation of serum AFP levels and a negative second-look laparotomy.

REFERENCES

Einhorn L H, Donahue J 1977 Cis-diamminodichloroplatinum, vinblastine and bleomycin combination chemotherapy in disseminated testicular cancer. Annals of Internal Medicine 87: 293
Forney J P 1978 Pregnancy following removal and chemotherapy of ovarian endodermal sinus tumour. Obstetrics and Gynecology 52: 361
Forney J P, Di Saia P J, Marrow C P 1975 Endodermal sinus tumour. A report of two sustained remissions treated postoperatively with a combination of actinomycin D, 5-fluorouracil and cyclophosphamide. Obstetrics and Gynecology 45: 186
Gallion H, van Nagell J R, et al 1979 Therapy of endodermal sinus tumour of the ovary. American Journal of Obstetrics and Gynecology 135: 447
Jimerson G K, Woodruff J D 1977 Ovarian extraembryonal teratoma. II. Endodermal sinus tumour mixed with other germ cell tumours. American Journal of Obstetrics and Gynecology 127: 302
Julian C G, Barrett J M, Richardson R L, Greco F A 1980 Bleomycin, vinblastine and cis-platinum in the treatment of advanced endodermal sinus tumour. Obstetrics and Gynecology 56: 396
Kurman R J, Norris H J 1976a Embryonal carcinoma of the ovary. A clinicopathologic entity distinct from endodermal sinus tumour resembling embryonal carcinoma of the adult testis. Cancer 38: 2420–2433
Kurman R J, Norris H J 1976b Endodermal sinus tumour of the ovary. A clinical and pathologic analysis of 71 cases. Cancer 38: 2404–2419
Piver M S, Lurain J 1979 Childhood ovarian cancers. New advances in treatment. New York State Journal of Medicine 79: 1196

Schiller W 1939 Mesonephroma ovarii. American Journal of Cancer 35: 1

Sell A, Sogaard H, Nargaard-Pedersen B 1976 Serum alpha-fetoprotein as a marker for the effect of postoperative radiation therapy and/or chemotherapy in 8 cases of ovarian endodermal sinus tumour. International Journal of Cancer 18: 574

Shrikhande S S, Sirsat M V 1975 Endodermal sinus tumour of the ovary (a study of 27 cases). Indian Journal of Cancer 151–157

Slayton R E, Hreshchyshyn M D, Silverberg S G et al 1978 Treatment of malignant ovarian germ cell tumours. Response to vincristine, dactinomycin and cyclophosphamide (preliminary report). Cancer 42: 390

Smith J P, Rutledge F 1975 Advances in chemotherapy for gynecologic cancer. Cancer 36: 669

Talerman A, Haije W G, Baggerman L 1978 Serum alphafetoprotein (AFP) in diagnosis and management of endodermal sinus (yolk sac) tumour and mixed germ cell tumour of the ovary. Cancer 41: 272–278

Teilum G 1959 Endodermal sinus tumours of the ovary and testis. Comparative morphogenesis of the so called mesonephroma ovarii (Schiller) and extraembryonic (yolk sac-allantoid) structures of the rat placenta. Cancer 12: 1092

Williams S, Slayton R, et al 1981 Response of malignant ovarian germ cell tumours to cis-platinum, vinblastine and bleomycin (PVB). Proceedings of Association of American Cancer Research and the American Society of Clinical Oncology 22: 463

12

Dysgerminoma

Introduction

Dysgerminomas are germ-cell tumours that are morphologically and ultrastructurally consistent with primordial germ cells and, in fact, arise from undifferentiated primordial germ cells. They are distinguished from other ovarian malignancies by their extreme radiocurability to low-dose radiation, their high cure rate and their propensity for para-aortic lymph node metastasis. Dysgerminoma is the most common malignant ovarian germ-cell tumour, being twice as common as endodermal sinus tumour (Norris & Jenson 1972). However, they only account for 1–2% of all ovarian tumours, and 3–5% of all ovarian malignancies. Most dysgerminomas occur in the second and third decade of life, with 75% occurring between the ages of 10 and 30. The median age is approximately 19–22 years.

The low survival rates reported previously, such as the 27.3% five-year survival rate by Mueller and associates in 1950, can be explained by four factors: (1) many of the early reports were prior to the megavoltage radiation era; (2) many of the early reports of dysgerminoma were in reality dysgerminoma admixed with the more aggressive embryonal carcinoma, endodermal sinus tumour or ovarian choriocarcinoma; (3) earlier reports used crude survival statistics as compared to the recent use of actuarial survival rates; and (4) dysgerminomas in earlier reports were diagnosed at a more advanced stage compared to the recent reports that indicate that 75% are stage I at diagnosis.

Symptoms

Pure dysgerminomas have no associated hormonal activity. However, in rare cases, patients with dysgerminoma admixed with gonadoblastoma may be virilised secondarily to hormonal stimulation by the surrounding stroma. Dysgerminomas have been reported to be associated with testicular feminisation, Turner syndrome and polycystic ovarian disease, each of which has associated genital abnormalities caused by the primary disease and not by the associated dysgerminoma. In contrast, most patients with dysgerminoma have normal sexual development. Symptoms include an abdominal mass or pelvic pain in over 50% of the patients. Fifteen to 20% of dysgerminomas occur during pregnancy or in the immediate postpartum period. This is in contrast to all ovarian malignancies in which approximately only 2–5% are associated with pregnancy. Dysgerminomas constitute 25–30% of all ovarian cancers coexistent with pregnancy. There is no known reason for this association. The previous reports of precocious puberty in patients with dysgerminoma probably represent human chorionic gonadotrophin (HCG) excretion by small areas of unrecognised ovarian choriocarcinoma in association with dysgerminoma, rather than the production of HCG by the dysgerminoma germ cells.

Pathology

Histologically, the dysgerminoma germ cells are easily recognisable. They may be associated, however, with syncitial giant cells which may contain histochemically demonstrable HCG (Ueda et al 1972). Granulomatous or lymphocytic infiltration are seen in most dysgerminomas, the amount of which correlates with prognosis. Of the 105 patients reported by Asadourian & Taylor (1969), 95 had a lymphocytic reaction which was marked in 15 of the patients. Moreover, 22 patients had granulomatous infiltration with histiocytic and giant cells. Of the 54 patients with only minimal lymphocytic infiltration, the mortality was 20%, compared to 6.7% (1) in the 15 patients with marked lymphocytic or granulomatous reaction. Increased mitotic activity and increased cellular atypia were also associated with prognosis and survival. Of the 30 patients with tumours with more than eight mitotic figures per five high-power fields, 23% died of dysgerminoma, compared to only 10% mortality rate in 58 patients with fewer mitotic figures.

Fifteen per cent of the patients died of dysgerminoma if there was marked cellular atypia, compared to a 9% mortality rate in cases with only minimal cellular atypia.

Conservative vs. non-conservative management of stage IA dysgerminoma

Since 15–30% of these young dysgerminoma patients will develop recurrence after conservative unilateral salpingo-oophorectomy, the decision for conservative management of clinical stage IA dysgerminoma is difficult. The situation is compounded by the fact that physicians are aware that most of the recurrences are radio-curable and therefore, adjuvant irradiation could be postponed until the recurrence develops. The unanswered question is whether nearly 100% cure rates are achievable by non-conservative surgery and whole abdominal irradiation in patients with stage IA dysgerminoma. Finally, the problem is further compounded because dysgerminoma is the only malignant ovarian germ-cell tumour that is frequently associated with bilateral ovarian involvement (15–25%) in the absence of metastasis. Seventy-five per cent of the Asadourian & Taylor (1969) patients had stage I dysgerminoma, 86% had stage IA, and 14% had stage IB. Of the patients with stage IB, two-thirds had visible malignancy in the contralateral ovary, whereas one-third had only occult microscopic involvement in the contralateral, normal appearing ovary.

Lucraft (1979) reported 12 stage IA patients whose ages ranged from 11 to 14 years. Four were given postoperative whole abdominal irradiation therapy and all survived without evidence of recurrence. Of the remaining eight patients, four developed recurrences, a 50% recurrence rate in those patients not receiving postoperative irradiation. These four patients were subsequently treated by whole abdominal irradiation and all survived without evidence of disease. Therefore, all 12 patients were surviving with no evidence of disease from three to more than 15 years whether given radiotherapy immediately, later for recurrence, or not at all.

This high recurrence rate is also seen in the Asadourian & Taylor study. Of their 46 patients treated by unilateral salpingo-oophorectomy for stage IA dysgerminoma, 22% (10) developed a recurrence and all were subsequently treated by radiation therapy. The overall survival rate for the 46 patients was 91%. This compares to the same 91% survival rate in their 11 patients treated by bilateral salpingo-oophorectomy without postoperative irradiation, but who indeed did have a lower initial recurrence rate of only 9%. However, these patients did not have preservation of future fertility. The 91% survival rate by conservative management is as good as the 86% survival rate in their patients treated by bilateral salpingo-oophorectomy plus radiation therapy, again with preservation of future fertility. At least 10 of their patients treated conservatively with unilateral salpingo-oophorectomy have had one or more successful pregnancies (Table 12.1).

Table 12.1 Unilateral dysgerminoma; recurrence and survival (Asadourian & Taylor 1969)

Management	No.	Recurrence %	(no.)	Survival
Unilateral oophorectomy	46	22%	(10)	91%
Bilateral oophorectomy	11	9%	(1)	91%
Oophorectomy plus radiation	14	14%	(2)	86%

Krepart and coauthors (1978) reported five patients treated by unilateral salpingo-oophorectomy who were observed without receiving postoperative radiotherapy. All were young and wanted to preserve their fertility. The difference in this report from that of previous reports is that these patients were preselected because of good prognostic factors. All had stage IA, well-differentiated dysgerminomas that measured less than 10 cm in diameter, were non-adherent to surrounding structures, and were well encapsulated. All were alive and well without evidence of recurrence from 36 to 212 months after surgical therapy. Three of these five patients subsequently had children. However, in seven additional patients with stage IA dysgerminoma measuring from 12.5 to 20 cm, all developed recurrences in 7 to 26 months after initial surgery (Table 12.2).

Table 12.2 Recurrent stage IA dysgerminoma (Krepart et al 1978)

Initial stage	Size of ovarian dysgerminoma	Area of recurrence	Time to recurrence (months)
IA	20 cm	Distant metastasis	7
IA	15 cm	Pelvis	8
IA	12.5 cm	Contralateral ovary	9
IA	23 cm	Distant metastasis	12
IA	18 cm	Abdomen	20
IA	15 cm	Abdomen	22
IA	15 cm	Abdomen	26

Our experience with the radiocurability of recurrent dysgerminoma is similar to that of Lucraft. All five patients. ages 10–17, had stage I dysgerminoma. Of the two patients receiving adjuvant whole abdominal and pelvic irradiation, neither developed recurrences. However, of the three patients that did not receive initial adjuvant radiotherapy for stage IA dysgerminoma, two developed recurrences. Both patients received radiation therapy to the sites of recurrence and are alive without evidence of disease for 9 and 10 years, respectively. All five patients are without evidence of disease from 2.5 to 12 years (Table 12.3). Four received either initial radiation therapy or radiation therapy for recurrence (Piver & Lurain 1979, Piver 1979).

Table 12.3 Stage I ovarian dysgerminoma (Piver & Lurain 1979)

Stage	Primary treatment	Recurrence	Treatment of recurrence	NED (years)
IA	Pelvic + abdominal RT	None	–	5[*]
IA	Pelvic + abdominal RT	None	–	2.5[+]
IA	None	Pelvic + abdominal	Pelvic + abdominal RT	10[+]
IB	None	None	–	12[+]
IC	None	Pelvis, abdominal, lungs	Pelvic, abdominal, lungs RT	9[+]

Conservative unilateral salpingo-oophorectomy should only be carried out for a pure dysgerminoma not admixed with the more aggressive endodermal sinus tumour, embryonal carcinoma or ovarian choriocarcinoma. The tumour should be no greater than 10 cm and preferably 8 cm or less in diameter and the retroperitoneal para-aortic lymph nodes and cytological washings should have no evidence of metastatic dysgerminoma. The contralateral, normal appearing ovary should be biopsied to rule out bilateral ovarian involvement which may be present in 5–25% of these tumours. Since the levels of the serum biological markers, serum beta-human chorionic gonadotrophin, and alpha-fetoprotein are not increased by pure dysgerminoma, these tumour markers should be obtained. An increase in either would suggest the admixture of other germ-cell tumours such as endodermal sinus tumour, embryonal carcinoma or ovarian choriocarcinoma. Finally, a pretherapy or postlaparatomy lymphangiogram should be performed in all cases (Table 12.4).

In contrast to the conservative approach of preserving possible

Table 12.4 Factors influencing conservative management of unilateral dysgerminoma

1. Young patient
2. Pure dysgerminoma
3. Tumour less than 8 cm, encapsulated, non-adherent
4. Retroperitoneal lymph nodes 'negative'
5. Pelvic and para-colic washings negative for malignant cells
6. Patient and family consent

future fertility by unilateral salpingo-oophorectomy is the report by Boyes et al (1979) on 25 dysgerminoma cases from 1938–1976, with a corrected five-year survival rate of 91%. There were no deaths in the 18 cases diagnosed since 1960 when their treatment method changed from unilateral salpingo-oophorectomy to hysterectomy and bilateral salpingo-oophorectomy followed by radiation therapy. They reported that this latter aggressive treatment, which has resulted in a 100% cure rate, negates the value of conservative management.

Although previous reports have advocated either conservative unilateral salpingo-oophorectomy, plus adjuvant pelvic and para-aortic nodal irradiation, a recent report by Creasman and co-authors (1979) may allow for improved survival as well as retention of future fertility. They reported five patients with stage IA anaplastic dysgerminoma treated by combination chemotherapy. They used the term anaplastic dysgerminoma because of the similarity to anaplastic seminoma of the testis, a recognised entity, that has the overall appearance of dysgerminoma but with an anaplastic appearance of the germ cells. Pleomorphism and increased mitotic activity are quite apparent. All five patients received combination chemotherapy consisting of methotrexate, actinomycin-D and chlorambucil (MAC) because of its efficacy against gestational ovarian choriocarcinoma (Table 12.5). No patient received radiation therapy and all received two or three five-day courses of MAC chemotherapy. They are all surviving 3, 20, 27, 30, and 36 months, respectively, without evidence of recurrence. Only further follow-

Table 12.5 MAC chemotherapy in stage IA anaplastic dysgerminoma (Creasman et al 1979)

Drug	Dose	Days
Methotrexate	12–15 mg/day	1–5
Actinomycin-D	0.5 mg/day	1–5
Chlorambucil	6–10 mg/day	1–5

Repeat every 2–4 weeks for 3 cycles

up will allow us to know whether adjuvant MAC chemotherapy without radiation therapy, does indeed result in long-term survival without recurrence, while preserving future fertility. If so, this would resolve the problem of conservative surgery vs. surgery plus postoperative irradiation.

Chemotherapy

There have been very few reports of the use of chemotherapy in metastatic or recurrent dysgerminomas. Krepart et al (1978) reported three patients receiving chemotherapy for recurrent dysgerminoma. One received cyclophosphamide and did not respond. The other two received actinomycin-D, 5-fluorouracil and cyclophosphamide, and both were in complete remission 16 and 15 months, respectively. Cohen & Goldsmith (1977) reported a patient with metastatic dysgerminoma who achieved a complete remission and possible cure four years after initial treatment with vincristine and bleomycin, followed by maintenance therapy with vincristine and methotrexate. Boyes et al (1979) treated two patients with cyclophosphamide for recurrence after surgery and radiation therapy. Both were in complete remission and free of disease 7 and 12 years later. Therefore, the reported effective chemotherapy for recurrent dysgerminoma not amenable to surgery or radiation therapy would be (1) cyclophosphamide; (2) vincristine plus bleomycin; (3) actinomycin-D, 5-fluorouracil and cyclophosphamide. An alternative choice of chemotherapy would be the effective combination chemotherapy regimens used in endodermal sinus tumour, embryonal carcinoma or immature teratoma; (1) vinblastine, bleomycin and cis-platinum (VBP) and (2) vincristine, actinomycin-D and cyclophosphamide (VAC).

Non conservative treatment: Surgery plus radiation therapy

All patients with stage IA–III dysgerminoma not treated conservatively should receive postoperative radiation therapy. If there is no evidence of para-aortic lymph node metastasis diagnosed by lymphangiography or at surgery, treatment should be to the whole abdomen and pelvis, 2500 to 3000 rads. If there is metastasis to the para-aortic lymph nodes, an additional 1500 rads should be

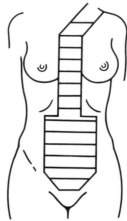

Fig. 12.1 Pelvic, abdominal, mediastinal and left supraclavicular radiation for dysgerminoma with para-aortic metastases.

delivered to a small field to include just the para-aortic lymph nodes. In such instances, the next higher chain of lymph nodes may be involved. Therefore, an additional 2500 rads prophylactic irradiation should be given to the mediastinum and left supraclavicular lymph nodes (Fig. 12.1).

REFERENCES

Asadourian L A, Taylor H B 1969 Dysgerminoma: An analysis of 105 cases. Obstetrics and Gynecology 33: 370

Boyes D A, Pankratz E, Galliford B W et al 1979 Experience with dysgerminomas at the cancer control agency of British Columbia. Gynecologic Oncology 6: 123

Cohen S M, Goldsmith M A 1977 Prolonged chemotherapeutic remission of metastatic ovarian dysgerminoma. Report of a case. Gynecologic Oncology 5: 299

Creasman W T, Fetter B F, Hammond C B, Parker R T 1979 Germ cell malignancies of the ovary. Obstetrics and Gynecology 53: 226

Krepart G, Smith J P, Rutledge F, Delclos L 1978 The treatment for dysgerminoma of the ovary. Cancer 41: 987

Lucraft H H 1979 A review of thirty-three cases of ovarian dysgerminoma emphasizing the role of radiotherapy. Clinical Radiology 30: 585

Mueller C W, Topkins P, Lapp W A 1950 Dysgerminoma of the ovary; Analysis of 427 cases. American Journal of Obstetrics and Gynecology 60: 153

Norris H J, Jenson R D 1972 Relative frequency of ovarian neoplasms in children and adolescents. Cancer 30: 713

Piver M S 1979 Unpublished data

Piver M S, Lurain J 1979 Childhood ovarian cancers. New York State Journal of Medicine 79: 1196

Ueda G, Hamanaka N, Hayakawak N, et al 1972 Clinical, histochemical, and biochemical studies of an ovarian dysgerminoma with trophoblasts and Leydig cells. American Journal of Obstetrics and Gynecology 114: 749

13

Ovarian choriocarcinoma and mixed germ-cell ovarian tumours

Introduction

Ovarian choriocarcinoma consists of an admixture of syncitiotrophoblasts and cytotrophoblasts similar to uterine choriocarcinoma. Ovarian choriocarcinoma can be a primary cancer resulting from an ovarian pregnancy (gestational choriocarcinoma), or not associated with an ovarian pregnancy (nongestational). More commonly, however, it is a secondary cancer, resulting from metastasis from a uterine choriocarcinoma. In either case, ovarian choriocarcinoma is associated with elevated human chorionic gonadotrophin levels, (HCG)

Gestational choriocarcinoma is extremely rare, and to date, only eight cases have been reported. For an ovarian choriocarcinoma to be considered gestational, it has to be presumed that it follows an ovarian pregnancy and there has to be proof that there was no prior uterine choriocarcinoma.

Nongestational ovarian choriocarcinoma is more common, and is usually associated with other germ-cell elements: dysgerminoma, endodermal sinus tumour, embryonal carcinoma or immature teratoma.

The earlier reports of the lack of response of ovarian choriocarcinoma to chemotherapy may be due, in part, to the fact that previous examples diagnosed as ovarian choriocarcinoma were, in reality, examples of the recently described embryonal carcinoma, which is also associated with elevated HCG. Therefore, the tumours did not respond to the chemotherapeutic agents used at that time for ovarian choriocarcinoma, namely, methotrexate or actinomycin-D.

Finally, ovarian choriocarcinoma may be one of the germ-cell

153

elements of a mixed germ-cell tumour which frequently contains areas of choriocarcinoma admixed with dysgerminoma, endodermal sinus tumour, embryonal carcinoma or immature teratoma.

Nongestational ovarian choriocarcinoma

Nongestational ovarian choriocarcinoma ususally occurs during the adolescent or premenarchial period. Like uterine choriocarcinoma, it is associated with elevated HCG levels. Wider and coauthors (1969) demonstrated the response of this rare tumour to combination chemotherapy consisting of methotrexate, actinomycin-D and chlorambucil (MAC) in four cases of nongestational ovarian choriocarcinoma admixed with other germ-cell elements. Three of the four patients had a complete response to chemotherapy and were without evidence of disease at last follow-up examination. The fourth died from her malignancy (Table 13.1).

Gerbie and coauthors (1975) reported treating eight cases of nongestational ovarian choriocarcinoma with either MAC chem-

Table 13.1 MAC chemotherapy of nongestational ovarian choriocarcinoma (Wider et al 1969)

Stage	Histology	Response	Status (months)
IV	Choriocarcinoma, dysgerminoma	Complete	NED (14)
IA	Choriocarcinoma, undifferentiated carcinoma	Complete	NED (46)
IIB	Choriocarcinoma, teratocarcinoma	Complete	NED (55)
IV	Choriocarcinoma	Partial	DOD (13)

NED = no evidence of disease   DOD = dead of disease

Table 13.2 Chemotherapy of nongestational ovarian choriocarcinoma (Gerbie et al 1975)

Pure choriocarcinoma			Mixed germ-cell tumours plus choriocarcinoma		
Stage	Chemotherapy	Status	Stage	Chemotherapy	Status
IV	Methotrexate	NED 11 years	III	MAC	NED 3 years
IA	Methotrexate Actinomycin-D	NED 6 years	IA	MAC	DOD 2.5 years
III	MAC	NED 1 year	IV	Methotrexate	DOD 1.5 years
IV	MAC	DOD 1 month	IV	MAC	DOD 6 months

otherapy, methotrexate, or methotrexate and actinomycin-D. All eight patients had elevated HCG levels. Of the four cases of pure ovarian choriocarcinoma, three survived without evidence of disease and one died of her malignancy. However, of the three patients with ovarian choriocarcinoma admixed with other germ-cell elements, only one survived and three died of their disease (Table 13.2).

Gestational ovarian choriocarcinoma

Of the eight reported cases of gestational ovarian choriocarcinoma (Acosta-Sison 1959, turner et al 1964, Patton & Goldstein 1973, Benjamin & Rorat 1978, Veridiano et al 1980), that of Patton & Goldstein was significant because it demonstrated the response of these tumours to chemotherapy and the long-term survival rates. Two of their patients had a complete response to methotrexate, with or without actinomycin-D, and both were alive with no evidence of disease, more than five years after treatment (Table 13.3).

Table 13.3 Chemotherapy of gestational choriocarcinoma (Patton & Goldstein 1973)

Stage	Elevated HCG	Chemotherapy	Response	Status (months)
IA	Yes	Methotrexate Actinomycin-D	Complete	NED (64)
IIB	Yes	Methotrexate	Complete	NED (66)
III	Yes	Actinomycin-D Methotrexate Triple chemotherapy	None	DOD (13)

Mixed germ-cell tumours

Kurman & Norris (1976) reported 30 cases of mixed germ-cell ovarian tumours. The patients's ages ranged from 5 to 33, with a median age of 16. Forty per cent of the patients were prepubertal. Precocious puberty, secondary to elevated HCG levels from elements of ovarian choriocarcinoma or embryonal carcinoma, occurred in one-third of the prepubertal girls. The 30 cases of mixed germ-cell ovarian tumours represented 8% of the germ-cell ovarian tumours seen at the Armed Forces Institute of Pathology and ranked fourth in incidence behind dysgerminoma (150), pure endodermal sinus tumour (71), malignant immature teratoma (50), mixed germ-cell tumours (30), and pure embryonal carcinoma (12). Histologically, dysgerminoma was the most common element seen, present in 70% of the 30 cases. Immature teratoma occurred in 53%, ovarian choriocarcinoma in 20%, and embryonal carcinoma in 16%. Endodermal sinus tumour and dysgerminoma accounted for one-third of the mixed germ-cell tumours and was the most common combination present.

Prognosis was dependent on the stage of the disease and, for patients with stage I mixed germ-cell ovarian tumours, was dependent on the germ-cell elements present and the maximum diameter of the tumour (Table 13.4).

Table 13.4 Mixed germ cell tumour: survival (Kurman & Norris 1976)

Stage	Patients	% Survival
I	18	50
II	4	75
III	4	0
IV	1	0

Of the patients with stage I mixed germ-cell tumours, only 25% (3/12) survived if more than one-third of the tumour consisted of endodermal sinus tumour, grade 3 immature teratoma or ovarian choriocarcinoma. This compared to a 100% (6/6) survival rate for those patients with tumours containing embryonal carcinoma, dys-

Table 13.5 Stage I mixed germ cell tumour; survival & prognosis factors (Kurman & Norris 1976)

Tumour size	Patients	% Survival
< 10 cm	4	100
> 10 cm	12	42
Dysgerminoma plus: grade 1 or 2 teratoma or embryonal carcinoma	3	100
< 1/3 Endodermal sinus, choriocarcinoma or grade 3 teratoma	3	100
> 1/3 Endodermal sinus, choriocarcinoma or grade 3 teratoma	12	25

germinoma or grade 1 or 2 immature teratoma. Of the patients with stage I malignant mixed germ-cell tumours in which the diameter of the tumour was actually known, 100% of the patients survived (4/4) if the tumour measured less than 10 cm in maximum diameter, compared to only 42% (5/12) for patients with tumours greater than 10 cm. Combining these two prognostic factors (histology and diameter), Kurman & Norris reported a 100% survival rate for patients with stage I mixed germ-cell tumours measuring less than 10 cm in maximum diameter and containing less than one-third ovarian choriocarcinoma, endodermal sinus tumour or grade 3 immature teratoma or did not contain these elements at all. None of the patients with tumours greater than 10 cm containing more than one-third ovarian choriocarcinoma, endodermal sinus tumour or grade 3 immature teratoma survived (Table 13.5).

Surgical and chemotherapeutic management of ovarian choriocarcinoma and mixed germ-cell tumours

Since ovarian choriocarcinoma is rarely bilateral and is associated with a specific tumour marker (beta-human chorionic gonadotrophin), conservative unilateral salpingo-oophorectomy allows for preservation of future fertility in young patients. Adjuvant chemotherapy with methotrexate, actinomycin-D and chlorambucil (MAC) is repeated until two consecutive normal beta-human chorionic gonadotrophin titres are achieved. Patients with stage IB–IV ovarian choriocarcinoma require maximal debulking surgery, followed by MAC chemotherapy.

The specific chemotherapy for mixed germ-cell ovarian tumours is less precise due primarily to the combinations of malignant elements present within the tumour. Patients with mixed germ-cell tumours consisting of more than one-third ovarian choriocarcinoma should receive methotrexate, actinomycin-D or MAC chemotherapy as part of their treatment. The effective chemotherapy for patients with mixed germ-cell tumours consisting of more than one-third endodermal sinus tumour, embryonal carcinoma or immature teratoma is vincristine, actinomycin-D and cyclophosphamide (VAC), or vinblastine, bleomycin and cis-platinum (VBP).

REFERENCES

Acosta-Sison H 1959 Ab initio choriocarcinoma. Obstetrics and Gynecology
13: 350
Benjamin F, Rorat E 1978 Primary gestational choriocarcinoma of the ovary.
American Journal of Obstetrics and Gynecology 131: 343
Gerbie M V, Brewer J I, Tamimi H 1975 Primary choriocarcinoma of the ovary.
Obstetrics and Gynecology 46: 720
Kurman R J, Norris H J 1976 Malignant mixed germ-cell tumours of the ovary.
A clinical and pathologic analysis of 30 cases. Obstetrics and Gynecology
48: 579
Patton G W, Goldstein D P 1973 Gestational choriocarcinoma of the tube and
ovary. Surgery, Gynecology and Obstetrics 137: 608
Turner B T, Douglass W M, Gladding T C 1964 Choriocarcinoma of the ovary.
Obstetrics and Gynecology 24: 918
Veridiano N P, Gal D, Delke I et al 1980 Gestational choriocarcinoma of the
ovary. Gynecologic Oncology 10: 235
Wider J A, Marshall J R, Bardin C W et al 1969 Sustained remissions after
chemotherapy for primary ovarian cancers containing choriocarcinoma. New
England Journal of Medicine 280: 1439

14

Primary ovarian carcinoids (insular carcinoid, trabecular carcinoid, strumal carcinoid and struma ovarii)

Introduction

Within the ovarian teratoma classification is a group of rare, germ-cell, monodermal or highly specialised, ovarian teratomas which consist of primary ovarian carcinoids and struma ovarii. There are four types of primary ovarian carcinoids. The most common type is the insular carcinoid which is similar to those tumours arising from the midgut or jejunum, the ileum and the appendix. Histologically, insular carcinoids consist of small groups of acini. The second most common type of primary ovarian carcinoid is the trabecular carcinoid which is similar to those tumours arising from the hindgut or foregut. These tumours are characterised by anastamosing trabecular columns or a ribbon-type pattern. The third type is the strumal carcinoid which consists of an admixture of trabecular carcinoid and thyroid tissue. The least common type is the carcinoid which develops within a Sertoli-Leydig cell tumour.

Primary ovarian carcinoids are of clinical interest because patients may initially have symptoms of the carcinoid syndrome (diarrhoea, cutaneous flush, wheezing, cardiac valvular disease), or symptoms of thyroid hyperfunction (tremor, tachycardia, heat intolerance, weight loss, muscle weakness or exopthalmus) and, therefore, they become important in the differential diagnosis of many disease entities. Primary ovarian carcinoids are important because of the necessity to differentiate them from carcinoids metastatic to the ovary, a disease which is almost uniformly fatal. This is in contrast to the excellent prognosis of primary ovarian carcinoids. Strumal ovarii patients may also initially have the symptoms of thyroid hyperfunction listed earlier.

The carcinoid syndrome occurs only with insular ovarian carcinoids or with metastatic carcinoids. The carcinoid syndrome symptoms are secondary to argyrophillic enterochromaffin (argentaffin) cells which synthesise and secrete serotonin, catecholamines and histamine which result in facial flushing, asthmatic symptoms, oedema of the head and neck and cardiac valvular disease (tricuspid insufficiency and pulmonary stenosis) (Satterlee et al 1970). Rarely, pedal oedema or hypertension occur. It was first thought that the chronic diarrhoea, cutaneous flush, cardiac valvular disease, skin rash and bronchial asthma were most often secondary to the secretion of excessive serotonin, the latter measured by urinary 5-hydroxyindole-acetic acid (5-HIAA). More recently, it has been reported that the cutaneous flush component of the carcinoid syndrome may be mediated by bradykinin (Mason & Melmon 1966).

Insular carcinoids

Most insular carcinoids are associated with teratomatous elements (respiratory and gastrointestinal epithelium or cartilage), but occasionally, they are the only element present. Insular carcinoids usually occur within a cystic teratoma or as a small part of a mature teratoma. Insular carcinoids occur most often in women 31–78 years of age, with the median age of 58 years. These carcinoids arise from argyrophillic enterochromaffin (argentaffin) cells which are primarily found in the gastrointestinal, biliary, pancreatic and respiratory epithelium. The argentaffin granules can be identified by ferric ferricyanide staining in approximately 80% of the cases. Histologically, insular carcinoids can be confused with granulosa cell tumours, Sertoli-Leydig cell tumours. Brenner tumours and gastrointestinal carcinoids metastatic to the ovary.

One-third of the insular carcinoids are associated with signs and symptoms of the carcinoid syndrome. In such instances, 5-HIAA is increased, but returns to normal within 24 hours of removal of the ovarian tumour. Insular carcinoids are always unilateral (FIGO stage IA) at the initial operation, and have no evidence of metastasis.

Robboy et al (1975) reported 48 cases of insular carcinoid, raising the total in the literature to 70 cases. The carcinoid syndrome occurred in 55% (15/27) of the patients with insular carcinoid measuring 4 cm in diameter or greater, compared to only a 5% (1/20) incidence if the insular carcinoid was less than 4 cm.

Follow-up data was available for 42 patients, all of whom originally had FIGO stage IA. Two patients subsequently died of recurrent insular carcinoid. The average follow-up was 6.9 years and the actuarial survival rate was 95% at five years and 88% at 10 years. Because of the excellent overall survival rate and the absence of bilateral ovarian involvement and metastatic implants at the initial operation, treatment in young patients desiring to retain future fertility is by unilateral salpingo-oophorectomy. Because so few of these tumours have recurred, there are few data regarding the effectiveness of radiation therapy or chemotherapy for recurrent primary ovarian carcinoids. Koven and coauthors (1968) did report a complete response and two-year survival after treatment with actinomycin-D. Since primary ovarian carcinoids are germ-cell ovarian tumours of teratomatous origin, treatment of the rare recurrences with vincristine, actinomycin-D and cylophosphamide (VAC), the current chemotherapy combination used for immature ovarian teratomas, would be appropriate.

The most important decision at the initial operation is to differentiate a primary ovarian carcinoid from a carcinoid metastatic to the ovary. Robboy et al (1974) reported 35 cases of carcinoid metastatic to the ovary and documented another 25 cases in their review of the literature. Carcinoids metastatic to the ovary account for less than 2% of all metastasis to the ovary, or less than 0.1% of all malignant ovarian tumours encountered at surgery. If the ovarian tumour is bilateral at initial operation, or if there is spread beyond the ovary, the diagnosis is almost certainly a carcinoid metastatic to the ovary. However, the findings of a unilateral primary ovarian carcinoid with associated teratomatous elements, and no evidence of metastasis at initial operation, is diagnostic of a primary ovarian carcinoid.

The carcinoid syndrome is present in 30 to 40% of insular carcinoids and carcinoids metastatic to the ovary. It is not present in the trabecular or strumal carcinoids. In cases of insular carcinoid, 5-HIAA decreases to normal within 24 hours of the removal of the ovarian tumour and remains normal. In carcinoids metastatic to the ovary, 5-HIAA does not return to normal rapidly after surgery and, by six months, it is still elevated in 75% of the cases.

Table 14.1 Primary ovarian carcinoid vs. carcinoid metastatic to the ovary
(Robboy et al 1974)

Characteristics	% in primary	% in metastatic
Unilateral	100	4
Teratomatous elements	76	0
Gastrointestinal primary	0	85
Peritoneal implants	0	92
Carcinoid syndrome	30–40	30–40
Syndrome & 5-HIAA recur after surgery	0	75
Recurrent carcinoid	4	96

Metastases are present in 92% of the metastatic carcinoids and in none of the primary ovarian carcinoids. The contralateral ovary is enlarged in 56% of the metastatic carcinoids and in 19% of the primary ovarian carcinoids. In the case of the primary ovarian carcinoids, this enlargement is secondary to dermoid cysts. Brenner tumours or mucinous cystadenomas and is not another primary ovarian carcinoid.

The contralateral ovary contains metastatic carcinoma in 96% of the metastatic carcinoids and in none of the primary ovarian carcinoids. Teratomatous tissue is present in 76% of the primary ovarian carcinoids and in none of the metastatic carcinoids. (Table 14.1) None of the patients with primary ovarian carcinoids were dead of their malignancy within one year of surgery, compared to 33% of those with metastatic carcinoids. At four years, none of the patients with primary ovarian carcinoids were dead of metastatic disease, compared to 75% of the patients with metastatic carcinoids. Recurrences developed in 4% of the primary ovarian carcinoids and 96% of the metastatic carcinoids (Koven et al 1968).

In those patients with carcinoid metastatic to the ovary, hysterectomy and bilateral salpingo-oophorectomy and resection of the primary intestinal carcinoid should be carried out.

Trabecular carcinoids

Histologically, trabecular carcinoids consist of anastamosing trabecular columns or a ribbon-like pattern. Trabecular carcinoids occur most often in women 24–74 years of age, with the median age of 47 years. Robboy, et al (1977) reported 18 cases of primary trabecular carcinoid of the ovary and could find only five additional cases in their review of the literature. None of the trabecular carcinoids were associated with the carcinoid syndrome and all were unilateral ovarian tumours without evidence of metastasis at the time of initial surgery. 5-HIAA was not elevated in the three patients in which it was measured.

Trabecular carcinoids have a weak reaction to ferric ferricyanide in contrast to a strongly positive reaction by the insular carcinoids. Trabecular carcinoids are distinguished from carcinoids metastatic to the ovary by unilateral ovarian involvement and the absence of metastasis. Only one patient in the Robboy et al series had endocrine hyperfunction, virilisation and endometrial hyperplasia, which was thought to be secondary to androgen and oestrogen production by the leutinised stromal cells seen in the periphery of the carcinoid.

The prognosis for patients with trabecular carcinoids is excellent. Of the 17 patients available for follow-up, only one died from trabecular carcinoid and the remaining 16 patients were alive for up to 15 years without recurrence, with a median follow-up of four years. Treatment for trabecular carcinoids is the same as that for insular carcinoids; unilateral salpingo-oophorectomy in the young patient desiring to retain future fertility.

Strumal carcinoids

In 1970, Scully coined the term strumal carcinoid for an ovarian tumour consisting of thyroid tissue intermixed with trabecular carcinoid. Previously, these tumours had been designated as malignant teratoma, malignant strumal ovarii, or rarely, papillary adenocarcinoma of the thyroid within a struma. Prior to the designation of strumal carcinoid, many of these tumours were included with the cases of malignant struma ovarii. Because of the non-ovarian tissue elements present within the tumour, strumal carcinoids are considered to be of teratomatous origin. They occur most often in women 21–77 years of age, with the median age of 53 years. Its identification as a primary ovarian carcinoid is made at initial operation by its unilateral ovarian involvement, without evidence of metastasis. Strumal carcinoid is not associated with the carcinoid syndrome. Rarely, strumal carcinoid has been associated with signs of virilisation secondary to leutinisation of the stromal cells. Occasionally, the thyroid tissue is functional. Robboy & Scully (1980) reported four strumal carcinoid patients with elevated biochemical parameters of thyroid function (elevated protein-bound iodine) and clinical evidence of functioning thyroid elements. Thyroid storm and hypothyroidism, respectively, developed in two patients after surgical removal of the ovarian strumal carcinoids.

Of the 50 cases of strumal carcinoid reported by Robboy & Scully, all were unilateral ovarian tumours at initial operation and none had biopsy-proven metastasis. Follow-up was available in 46 of the patients and one had died of recurrent strumal carcinoid. Because of its low recurrence rate, unilateral salpingo-oophorectomy in the young patient desiring to retain future fertility is the treatment of choice.

Struma ovarii

The term struma ovarii is reserved for those ovarian tumours where more than 50% of the tumour consists of thyroid tissue. They primarily occur within a benign cystic teratoma. Struma ovarii are uncommon and account for less than 2% of all ovarian teratomas. They should not be confused with the benign cystic teratoma in which a small foci of thyroid tissue is present. Thyroid tissue does occur in 7–15% of teratomas.

Struma ovarii have occurred in adolescents and in the very elderly, but most often they occur between 50 and 60 years of age. Less than 5% of struma ovarii have evidence of thyroid function. Woodruff & Markley (1957) reported metastasis of a struma ovarii to the lung. The patient was well 11 years after the pulmonary metastasis was treated with [131]I. In 1966, Woodruff et al reported 19 cases of struma ovarii. One patient developed metastasis to the liver which was treated successfully by radiation therapy to the liver.

Kempers et al (1970), reported 25 patients with struma ovarii, in eight of whom, there was evidence of hyperfunctioning thyroid tissue with signs and symptoms of hyperthyroidism. In five patients with clinical evidence of hyperthyroidism, a simultaneous cervical goiter was also present, making it difficult to establish the site of origin of the hyperfunctioning thyroid tissue. Nine of the 25 patients had significant amounts of ascites, in conjunction with a pelvic tumour, four of which were malignant struma ovarii. Only 11 of the 25 patients were asymptomatic, i.e., without ascites and signs of hyperfunctioning thyroid tissue. Five of the 25 tumours had undergone malignant change. Treatment of four of these malignant struma ovarii patients consisted of bilateral salpingo-oophorectomy and in one patient, a unilateral salpingo-oophorectomy was performed, with preservation of the normal appearing contralateral ovary. Only one patient had metastasis at initial operation but metastasis did occur subsequently in two other patients. These metastatic lesions were successfully treated by high-dose radioiodine. Four of the five patients with malignant struma ovarii were alive 5 to 21 years after treatment.

Unilateral salpingo-oophorectomy is the treatment of choice in young struma ovarii patients who desire future fertility. Postoperatively, body scanning, after administration of ^{131}I, should be carried out to be certain that there are no functioning metastatic struma ovarii present that require adjuvant therapy.

Summary

Insular carcinoid, trabecular carcinoid, strumal carcinoid and struma ovarii are all associated with a good prognosis. For those younger patients desiring to retain future fertility, treatment is by unilateral salpingo-oophorectomy. Since the majority of these tumours occur in patients past the childbearing age, treatment is by hysterectomy and bilateral salpingo-oophorectomy in most instances. For the rare patient with a recurrent primary ovarian carcinoid that is not amenable to complete surgical resection, vincristine, actinomycin-D and cyclophosphomide (VAC) chemotherapy, as used in patients with immature ovarian teratoma, would appear to be justified.

Patients with recurrent or metastatic struma ovarii are successfully treated by radioiodine. Radioisotope uptake, however, in metastatic struma ovarii may be enhanced by thyroidectomy, followed by complete oblation of any remaining cervical tissue with radioiodine.

REFERENCES

Kempers R D, Dockerty M B, Hoffman D L, Bartholomew L G 1970 Struma ovarii-ascitic, hyperthyroid and asymptomatic syndromes. Annals of Internal Medicine 72: 883–893
Koven B J, Collinger M R, Nadel M S 1968 Response to actinomycin-D of malignant carcinoid arising in an ovarian teratoma. American Journal of Obstetrics and Gynecology 101: 267
Mason D T, Melmon K L 1966 New understanding of the mechanism of the carcinoid flush. Annals of Internal Medicine 65: 1344

Robboy S J, Scully R E 1980 Strumal carcinoid of the ovary: An analysis of 50 cases of a distinctive tumor composed of thyroid tissue and carcinoid. Cancer 46: 2019–2034

Robboy S J, Norris H J, Scully R E 1975 Insular carcinoid primary in the ovary. A clinicopathologic analysis of 48 cases. Cancer 36: 404

Robboy S J, Scully R E, Norris H J 1974 Carcinoid metastatic to the ovary. A clinicopathologic analysis of 35 cases. Cancer 33: 798–811

Robboy S J, Scully R E, Norris H J 1977 Primary trabecular carcinoid of the ovary. Obstetrics and Gynecology 49: 202–207

Satterlee W G, Serpick A, Bianchine J R 1970 The carcinoid syndrome: Chronic treatment with para-chlorophenylalanine. Annals of Internal Medicine 72: 919–921

Scully R E 1970 Recent progress in ovarian cancer. Human Pathology 1: 73

Woodruff J D, Markley R L 1957 Struma ovarii. Obstetrics and Gynecology 9: 707

Woodruff J D, Rauh J T, Markley R L 1966 Ovarian struma. Obstetrics and Gynecology 27: 194–201

15

Granulosa cell tumours

Introduction

Granulosa cell tumours account for 3–10% of malignant ovarian tumours and 80% of hormonally active ovarian tumours. Granulosa-theca cell and Sertoli-Leydig cell ovarian tumours are referred to as sex-cord stromal tumours because they were originally thought to be derived from the sex-cord of the embryonic gonad. To date, their exact derivation remains speculative. Granulosa tumours can contain granulosa cells, theca cells, fibroblasts, Sertoli cells and/or Leydig cells, alone or in combination. They are classified into four categories: (1) female cell type including granulosa cell tumours, thecomas, granulosa-theca cell tumours, and thecoma-fibroma tumours (the designation thecoma-fibroma is used because in many instances a distinction between thecomas and fibromas is impossible); (2) male type, including Sertoli cell tumours, Leydig cell tumours, and Sertoli-Leydig cell tumours (previously referred to as arrhenoblastoma or androblastoma); (3) male and female cell types, including gynandroblastoma (granulosa and Sertoli or Leydig cells); and (4) unclassified sex-cord stromal tumours which include sex-cord tumours with annular tubules, and sclerosing stromal tumours.

Granulosa cell tumours are composed of granulosa cells alone, or combined with cells derived from the theca interna or externa. Granulosa cell tumours or those with theca cell elements (granulosa-theca) are included together regarding therapy because the prognosis depends entirely on the granulosa cells and not on the presence or absence of theca cells.

Histological diagnosis

Although sex-cord stromal tumours (granulosa-theca and Sertoli-Leydig) are capable of steroid production with resultant feminising or virilising symptoms, the specific diagnosis (male or female type) is based on histological criteria regardless of the type of hormonal production. The malignant potential of sex-cord stromal tumours has not been determined, although most are considered to have low malignant potential. The difficulty in determining the malignant potential of granulosa-theca cell tumours results because they are composed of cells with the appearance of the normal granulosa layer of the developing follicle, and therefore, frequently lack the common characteristics of anaplasia: cellular atypism, abnormal mitosis and hyperchromatism. The difficulty in determining what percentage of granulosa-theca cell tumours will act in a malignant manner (recur or metastasise) is compounded by the variation in histological criteria used for their diagnosis. Thus, many reports include, along with clearly diagnosed granulosa-theca cell tumours, many tumours which are misdiagnosed as granulosa-theca cell tumours. Stenwig et al (1979) documented this tendency for variations in the diagnosis of granulosa-theca cell tumours among pathologists. They reviewed 177 patients who had a previous diagnosis of granulosa-theca cell tumours, and 23% (41) of the cases had to be deleted from the study because of a revision in diagnosis on rereview (Table 15.1). Clearly, the results reported by Stenwig and coauthors would have been significantly different with the inclusion of 41 non-granulosa-theca cell tumours. Simi-

Table 15.1 Revision from original diagnosis of granulosa cell tumour (Stenwig et al 1979)

Revised diagnosis	Number
Adenocarcinoma	9
Thecoma	8
Androblastoma	7
Unclassified sex-cord tumour	3
Carcinoid tumour	3
Lymphoma	3
Hilus cell tumour	2
Sex-cord tumour with annular tubules	2
Poorly differentiated carcinoma	2
Brenner tumour	1
Adenocarcinoma metastatic to the ovary	1
Total	41

larly, in an analysis of 307 granulosa-theca cell tumours from the Ovarian Tumor Registry of Johns Hopkins University, by five 'leading pathologists,' the difficulty in assessing the malignant potential of these tumours was highlighted by their statement that 'accurate prognosis from the morphology of the functioning ovarian tumours (granulosa-theca) should be considered as no more reliable than an educated guess'; if the expertise of the Ovarian Tumor Registry is associated with certain inaccuracies, how reliable must be considered reports from the average general pathologist who is rarely confronted by these unusual ovarian tumours (Novak et al 1971)?

Norris & Taylor (1968) used the most rigid histological criteria for the diagnosis of granulosa-theca cell tumours, which may account, in part, for their exceedingly good results compared to other studies. Norris & Taylor only included as granulosa-theca cell tumours those with a nuclear groove (coffee bean nuclei) which is characteristic of sex-cord stromal tumours in general. The nuclear groove is secondary to a folded appearance of the nuclear membrane (Fig. 15.1). Moreover, to remove the possibility of including non-granulosa-theca cell tumours which may mimic granulosa-theca cell tumours histologically, they excluded tumours that had ducts or mucin as demonstrated by mucicarmen stain as

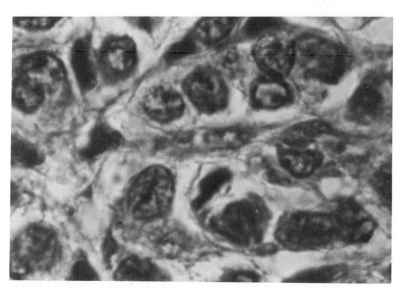

Fig. 15.1 High power view of a granulosa cell tumour demonstrating characteristic nuclear groove or coffee bean nuclei

seen in ovarian adenocarcinoma, or acinar structures as seen in ovarian carcinoids.

A majority of granulosa-theca cell tumours, 50–60%, have a characteristic rosette arrangement of the granulosa-theca cells referred to as Call-Exner bodies, and are similar to those seen in the graffian follicle. Areas of small gland formation in ovarian adenocarcinomas may give the appearance of rosette formation, resulting in the misinterpretation of Call-Exner bodies, and thus, a diagnosis of granulosa-theca cell tumour. Ovarian adenocarcinomas lack, however, the nuclear groove characteristic of sex-cord stromal tumours. Norris & Taylor observed that most ovarian tumours diagnosed as granulosa-theca cell tumours that have marked cellular atypia, marked pleomorphism, mucin production, or atypical mitosis are not granulosa-theca cell tumours, but rather are poorly differentiated carcinoma.

Histological criteria and prognosis

Granulosa-theca cell tumours have been subclassified into three main histological patterns: (1) follicular, (2) trabecular or insular, and (3) diffuse. Follicular granulosa-theca cell tumours are well differentiated and either micro or macrofollicular in character, with the microfollicular pattern characterised by the presence of Call-Exner bodies. The trabecular or insular type are well to intermediate in differentiation and do not form Call-Exner bodies. The diffuse (formerly sarcomatoid) are poorly differentiated and are often confused with thecomas. The theca cells are distinguished within a granulosa-theca cell tumour by the use of a reticulum stain; with the reticulum surrounding the individual theca cells, but with little or no reticulum surrounding the granulosa cells.

Histological patterns, capsular invasion, lymphatic invasion, cellular atypia and mitosis have been evaluated as possible prognosticators of recurrence and survival in patients with granulosa-theca cell tumours. The diffuse pattern, previously thought to have a worse prognosis as compared to follicular or trabecular patterns, was present in 50% of the 118 cases of granulosa-theca cell tumours reported by Stenwig and coauthors (1979). However, it had no influence on prognosis. Norris & Taylor (1968) also found no relationship between histological pattern and the persistence of granulosa-theca cell tumours. These authors also evaluated capsular invasion, lymphatic invasion, cellular atypia and mitosis in relation to the recurrence of persistence of granulosa-theca cell tumours. Of the 88 granulosa-theca cell tumours, eight had histological evidence of capsular invasion, and the tumour persisted in four of these patients. However, all four patients had granulosa-theca cell tumours which extended beyond the ovary at initial operation, and accounted for the persistence of the tumour, rather than the criteria of capsular invasion. In contrast, all four patients with only microscopic evidence of capsular invasion were without evidence of recurrence for over six years. Of the seven patients with lymphatic invasion, two had persistence of their tumour (29%). Moreover, the degree of mitosis or cellular atypia did not correlate with persistence of tumour in the Norris & Taylor series. In the Stenwig report, mortality did increase with the degree of mitosis. The difference in survival was statistically significant for three or more mitosis per 10 high-power field, compared to less than three mitosis per 10 high-power field. Moreover, mortality increased with increased cellular atypism between no atypism and 2+ atypism. The explanation for the dichotomy in the two series as related to mitosis, cellular atypism, and survival is unclear. Moreover, since there is little agreement among most authors regarding these histological criteria and persistence of granulosa-theca cell tumours, the use of such criteria in therapeutic decision making is not possible at this time.

Steroid production

McNatty and coauthors (1979) demonstrated that granulosa cell, theca cell and ovarian stroma cell tumours can produce oestrogen (oestradione, oestradiol), androgens (androstenedione, testosterone) and progesterone. In earlier reports, the production of oestrogens by granulosa cells was not well documented. However, by using specific antisera, Kurman and coauthors (1979) also demonstrated that granulosa cells specifically can produce testosterone, oestradiol, and progesterone. Theca cells, however, are responsible for the major production of oestrogens.

After removal of granulosa-theca cell tumours, oestrogen production usually returns to normal. McCormick & Riddick (1976) collected 10 reports of patients with granulosa-theca cell tumours who had preoperative and postoperative 24-hour urinary assays

Table 15.2 Granulosa-theca cell tumours: 24 hour urinary oestrogens (McCormack & Riddick 1976)

Author	Preoperative values μg/24 hours	Postoperative values μg/24 hours
Beisher	113	6
	64	10
	13	0
Brown	25	7
Fathalia	17.8	0
Procope	4.6	4.5
Woodruff	21	7
Targett	17.1	1.4
Besche	448	57.1

for oestrogens. Nine of the 10 patients had a significant decrease in the urinary oestrogen excretion after the removal of the granulosa-theca cell tumour (Table 15.2).

Seventy-five per cent of granulosa-theca cell tumours are endocrinologically active: feminising (oestrogenic) or virilising (androgenic). Symptoms related to this hyperoestrogenic state were reviewed from the literature by Anikwue and coauthors (1978) on 241 granulosa-theca cell tumour patients. They reported that 35% had postmenopausal bleeding, 14% menometrorrhagia and 3% breast changes. The increased oestrogen production is also reflected in the endometrial changes. In their review of 129 granulosa-theca cell tumour patients, Anikwue and coauthors reported that 62% had endometrial hyperplasia, 13% endometrial adenocarcinoma and only 20% had normal endometrium. Cystic hyperplasia was the most common, and adenomatous hyperplasia occurred less frequently. Similarly, Norris & Taylor (1968) had endometrium available from 77 of their patients with granulosa-theca cell tumours, and 9% had adenocarcinomas, 5% atypical hyperplasia, 17% adenomatous hyperplasia, and 13% cystic hyperplasia (Table 15.3).

Table 15.3 Endometrial findings in the presence of granulosa-theca cell tumours (Norris & Taylor 1968)

Histology	Granulosa	Granulosa-theca	Thecoma	Total %
Adenocarcinoma	6	15	8	9
Atypical hyperplasia	6	5	5	5
Adenomatous hyperplasia	22	15	16	17
Cystic hyperplasia	50	30	31	35
Other	–	–	–	33

Virilising symptoms included either hirsutism, oligomenor-rhoea, or amenorrhoea, and occurred in 3% of the patients. Finally, granulosa-theca cell tumours can produce progesterone. Lomax et al (1977) were the first to report markedly elevated levels of serum progesterone from a metastatic granulosa-theca cell tumour. These elevated levels returned to normal after a complete response to chemotherapy.

Cystic variety of granulosa cell tumours

Norris & Taylor (1969) described the first report of virilisation associated with an unusual cystic variety of granulosa-theca cell tumour. The unusual feature of the tumour was the extensive degree of cystic change which is suggestive of a serous cystadenoma. The original two patients in their study were each 15 years of age. Later, they reviewed 150 gonadal stromal tumours and found an additional seven cases of cystic granulosa-theca cell tumour. One of the seven patients had virilisation documented by severe hirsutism. All cystic granulosa-theca cell tumours occurred in young patients and proved clinically benign.

Juvenile granulosa-theca cell tumours

Scully (1977) described a distinctive form of granulosa-theca tumour which he named juvenile granulosa-theca cell tumour, and which occurs almost always in the first two decades. It is characterised by a macrofollicular or diffuse pattern of growth and often with extensive leutinisation of the granulosa, the theca cells, and hyperchromatic nuclei which gives this tumour a more unusual appearance than justified by its clinical behaviour. Roth and coauthors (1979) reported three cases, ages 7.5, 10, and a newborn female. The 7.5 year old presented with precocious pseudopuberty and the oestrogenic effect was confirmed by elevated serum levels of oestradiol which fell to a low level after removal of the tumour. The malignant potential of these tumours is unknown, but it is probably similar to granulosa-theca cell tumours in general.

Survival

Because of the variations in histological criteria for diagnosing granulosa-theca cell tumours, it is difficult to compare survival

Table 15.4 Granulosa-theca cell tumours: survival rates (Norris & Taylor 1968)

Histology	No. of patients	% Actuarial survival 5 Years	10 Years
Granulosa	44	97	93
Granulosa-theca	44	97	93
Thecoma	99	100	98

data from institution to institution. Using strict criteria (presence of nuclear grooves, absence of ducts, acinar structures and mucin), Norris & Taylor (1968), from the Armed Forces Institute of Pathology, reported the best survival rates to date, with 97% and 93% of the patients surviving 5 and 10 years, respectively, for pure granulosa cell tumours or granulosa-theca cell tumours. Norris & Taylor calculated survival rates by including only deaths from granulosa-theca cell tumours and excluding patients who died postoperatively, or who died of causes other than granulosa-theca cell tumours (Table 15.4). Their excellent 5 and 10-year actuarial survival rates (97% and 93%) included all stages (I, II, and III), though most patients had stage IA disease. The low rate of recurrence in the Norris & Taylor report was not related to the type of treatment: 72% of the patients were treated by unilateral salpingo-oophorectomy (with or without hysterectomy), and only 28% had bilateral salpingo-oophorectomy and hysterectomy as initial treatment. Only a few patients received adjuvant postoperative radiation therapy. They, as other authors, noted that long-term follow-up was necessary since many deaths from granulosa-theca cell tumours occur after five years, and may occur as late as 20 to 30 years after initial operation.

Stenwig and coauthors (1979) reported on 118 granulosa-theca celltumour patients from the Norweeian Radium Hospital. They included all deaths, using the life table method for calculating length of survival. Of their 91 stage I patients, the relative survival rate for 5, 10 and 15 years was 92%, 86% and 93% respectively. The survival rate decreased significantly to 76%, 61%, and 27% at 5, 10 and 15 years from the 21 stage II patients, and only 20% of the five stage III patients survived five years. Comparing stage I patients treated by surgery alone to those treated by surgery and postoperative pelvic irradiation, there was no significant improvement by the addition of postoperative radiation therapy. Moreover, when only deaths from granulosa-theca cell tumours were used as the basis for survival, the difference in five-year survival rates was significantly better for those treated by surgery alone

174

compared to those treated by surgery and postoperative radiation therapy. Only the report of Schwartz & Smith (1976) demonstrated a beneficial effect of postoperative radiation therapy in granulosa-theca cell tumours. However, this effect was seen when stages I, II and III were compared collectively, while the effect on stage I patients alone was not assessed.

Evans and coauthors (1980) reported 118 patients with granulosa-theca cell tumours treated at the Mayo Clinic from 1910 to 1972. Of the 93 stage I patients, 10 developed recurrences (10.7%), and 7 died (7.4%).

Using crude cumulative survival rates, Bjorklund & Pettersson (1980) reported survival rates of 91% at 5 years and 81% at 10 years in their study of 224 stage IA patients from the Radiumhemmet. Survival rates of the 224 stage IA patients, using only deaths from granulosa-theca cell tumours, were not reported.

It is clear from these four series that five-year survival rates (97% and 92% and 91%) for most localised granulosa theca cell tumours are excellent, but that they vary with the method of calculating survival rates. The method used for calculating survival rates is significant because many of these patients died from diseases other than granulosa-theca cell tumours. The 10-year survival rates reported by Norris & Taylor, Stenwig et al, and Bjorkholm & Pettersson were 93%, 86% and 81%, respectively. A mortality rate of nearly 20% from primarily localised granulosa-theca cell tumours would indicate the need for adjuvant therapy. However, since most reports, other than Norris & Taylor, include deaths from all cases, the actual 10-year mortality rate from localised granulosa-theca cell tumours is difficult to calculate. Therefore, the need for adjuvant radiation therapy or chemotherapy remains unclear. Moreover, to date, there are no reports of improved survival by using adjuvant therapies.

Chemotherapy for recurrent or metastatic granulosa-theca cell tumours

Since granulosa-theca cell tumours are of a low-grade malignant potential, recurrences are rare, and there are few reports regarding the use of chemotherapy (Lomax et al 1977, Schwartz & Smith 1976, Lusch et al 1978, Malkasian et al 1974, Barlow et al 1973, DiSaia et al 1978). As seen in Table 15.5, the majority of patients were treated with single agent chemotherapy (melphalan, adria-

Table 15.5 Chemotherapy of granulosa-theca cell tumours

Drug(s) & authors	Response complete	partial	none	Duration of response (months)
Melphalan				
Schwartz & Smith 1976	0	1	8	14
Lomax et al 1977	1	0	0	12+
Lusch et al 1978	1	0	0	19+
Malkasian et al 1974	0	0	2	–
Total	2	1	10	
Adriamycin				
*Barlow et al 1973	1	0	0	10
Di Saia et al 1978	1	0	0	12
ACFUCY				
Schwartz & Smith 1976	2	0	0	35+, 27+
Triethylenethiophosphoramide				
Schwartz & Smith 1976	0	0	4	–
Cyclophosphamide				
Malkasian et al 1974	0	3	9	3m+
5-Fluorouracil				
Malkasian et al 1974	0	1	2	3m+

* Plus bleomycin

mycin, triethylenethiophosphoramide, cyclosphosphamide and 5-fluorouracil). Of the 10 patients treated with melphalan, only three responded. However, two had complete responses and continue to survive without evidence of recurrent disease at 12 and 19 months, respectively. Two additional patients treated with actinomycin-D, 5-fluorouracil and cyclophosphamide (ACFUCY) had complete response, and both were without evidence of disease at 35 and 27 months, respectively. Of the two patients who received adriamycin (one with bleomycin), both had complete responses, but subsequently relapsed. Therefore, although reports of chemotherapy in patients with granulosa-theca cell tumours are few, the best reports to date are those including single agent melphalan, adriamycin, or the ACFUCY combination.

Thecomas

The diagnosis of a benign thecoma is based on finding spindle or oval cells with reticulum fibres surrounding individual theca cells, and the demonstration of intracellular lipid. The diagnosis of a malignant thecoma is more difficult. In 1979, Waxman and co-authors reviewed all of the reported cases of 'thecomas,' and stated that,

'Cases previously reported in the world literature as malignant the-comas were analyzed, and most of them were considered inade-quately documented; indeed most of them were probably either sarcomatoid granulosa cell tumors, stromal sarcomas, or fibrosar-comas. If a thecoma ever becomes malignant, the tumor cells dedifferentiate so that they cannot be recognized any longer as theca cells; instead, they proliferate as a stromal sarcoma or fibro-sarcoma. It is proposed therefore that the term 'malignant thecoma' not be used. On the other hand, very rare malignant ovarian stromal tumors do exist, consisting of undifferentiated stromal cells, fibroblasts, theca cells, which can show evidence of hormonal activ-ity.' (Waxman et al 1979)

This assessment of the malignant potential of thecomas is probably true.

Of the 99 thecomas reported by Norris & Taylor (1968), the 5- and 10-year actuarial survival rates were 100% and 98% respec-tively. Moreover, it is probable that the one death from a 'malig-nant thecoma,' was not a thecoma, since histologically, it was a low-grade fibrosarcoma that was hormonally inactive. Similarly, of the 82 patients with thecoma reported by Evans and coauthors (1980), there were no recurrences.

Thecomas occur primarily in peri- and postmenopausal women and are normally associated with oestrogenic activity. They are the most common of the functional ovarian tumours. In a litera-ture review of 225 cases by Anikwue et al (1978), 16% presented with menometrorrhagia, 8.4% of oligomenorrhoea, 30% post-menopausal bleeding and 4% were detected during pregnancy. In 150 cases where findings were recorded, abdominal swelling was present in 10% and a pelvic mass in 29%. Of the 72 cases where endometrium was available for evaluation, 17% had endometrial adenocarcinoma, 37% endometrial hyperplasia and 46% normal endometrium. There were no cases of hirsutism or other signs of virilisation recorded.

Unclassified sex-cord stromal tumours

Sclerosing ovarian stromal tumour

In 10% of sex-cord stromal tumours, it is impossible to tell if the cells are typical of the male or female gonad. One rare distinct subtype is the sclerosing ovarian stromal tumour, originally described by Chalvardjian & Scully (1973). It was so named because of its characteristic feature of cellular areas undergoing collagenous sclerosis. They originally described 10 tumours which appeared to be derived from ovarian stroma, but which had features sufficiently distinctive to separate them from fibromas and thecomas. The mean age at occurrence was 28 compared to ovarian stromal tumours which occur primarily in peri- and postmenopausal females. However, the most common symptom was menstrual irregularity which is probably indicative of hormonal activity, although the authors stated that none of the 10 tumours were hormonally active. In contrast, Damjanov et al (1975) reported the first case of sclerosing ovarian stromal tumour with detailed endocrinological studies which demonstrated the tumour was hormonally active and secreted oestrogen and androgens. To date, there have been no reports of a malignant sclerosing ovarian stromal tumour.

Sex-cord tumour with annular tubules (SCTAT)

In 1970, Scully described a distinct subtype of ovarian stromal tumour characterised by simple and complex ring-shaped tubules which had patterns intermediate between granulosa-theca cell tumours and a Sertoli cell tumour, and which resembled a gonadoblastoma except for the absence of germ cell components. SCTAT tumours are thought to produce oestrogens, since there are rare reports of cystic hyperplasia of the endometrium and isosexual precosity associated with these tumours. They are frequently associated with the Peutz-Jeghers syndromes. In 1980, Hart and coauthors documented the malignant potential of SCTAT tumours. Two of their six cases developed metastasis at 7.5 years and 10.5 years after the initial operation, respectively. Because of the histological and ultrastructural similarity to granulosa-theca cell tumours, they proposed that SCTAT tumours should be classified as an unusual subtype of granulosa-theca cell tumour in which annular formations and accumulations of basement membrane are prominent. Moreover, they pointed out that patients with SCTAT tumours should be treated similarly to patients with granulosa-theca cell tumours since their clinical behaviour with late recurrences were comparable.

Gynandroblastoma

Gynandroblastomas of the ovary are sex-cord stromal tumours containing both granulosa and either Sertoli or Leydig cells. Since the original description by Meyer in 1930, there have been only occasional reports of gynandroblastoma. These rare tumours may be associated with either feminising or virilising symptoms. Only rare reports of death from gynandroblastomas have been reported and, therefore, their malignant potential and treatment is generally similar to granulosa-theca cell tumours.

Treatment of granulosa-theca cell tumours

It is clear that those tumours which have minimal or no malignant potential — thecomas, juvenile granulosa-theca cell tumours, cystic variety of granulosa cell tumours, and sclerosing tumours of the ovary — should be treated conservatively by unilateral salpingo-oophorectomy in the young patient desiring to retain future fertility. However, the treatment of patients with granulosa-theca cell tumours is less clear because: (1) the malignant potential has never been established, (2) authors vary in the histological criteria for the diagnosis of granulosa-theca cell tumours, and (3) methods for calculating survival rates in patients with granulosa-theca cell tumours vary from author to author.

Treatment of granulosa-theca cell tumours depends on: (1) stage of disease, (2) presence or absence of bilateral ovarian granulosa-theca cell tumours, (3) age of the patient, (4) pathologist's criteria for diagnosing granulosa-theca cell tumours, and (5) status of the endometrium. The median age of patients with granulosa-theca cell tumours is 45–55 years of age, and only 5% occur in prepubertal girls. Most granulosa-theca cell tumours are stage IA at initial operation, with less than 5% bilateral (stage IB) at initial operation. As previously stated, the malignant potential of the granulosa-theca cell tumours cannot be determined by the usual morphological criteria because of the frequent absence of such criteria for anaplasia, cellular atypia, abnormal or frequent mitosis, and hyperchromatic nuclei. Since approximately 95% of granulosa-theca cell tumours are unilateral at initial operation, the 5- and 10-year actuarial survival rates have been reported as 97% and 93%, respectively; and since there is no documentation that adjuvant or postoperative radiation therapy or chemotherapy improves survival, conservative unilateral salpingo-oophorectomy in the young patient desiring to retain future fertility would be the treatment of choice. For patients not desiring future fertility, hysterectomy and bilateral salpingo-oophorectomy should be performed. In cases of stage II and III granulosa-theca cell tumours with small residual disease, postoperative whole abdominal irradiation, as documented by Schwartz & Smith (1976), may be beneficial. Finally, for patients with large residual metastatic disease or recurrent disease not amenable to surgery or radiation therapy, complete remissions or possible long-term cures have been reported with single agent melphalan and combination actinomycin-D, 5-fluorouracil and cyclophosphamide, whereas complete remissions, but not long-term cures, have been reported with adriamycin.

REFERENCES

Anikwue C, Dawood M Y, Dramer E 1978 Granulosa and theca cell tumors. Obstetrics and Gynecology 51: 214–220

Barlow J J, Piver M S, et al 1973 Adriamycin and bleomycin alone or in combination in gynecologic cancers. Cancer 32: 735

Bjorkholm E, Pettersson F 1980 Granulosa-cell and theca-cell tumors. A clinical picture and long-term outcome for the Radiumhemmet series. Acta obstetrica et gynecologica scandanavica 59: 361–365

Chalvardjian A, Scully R 1973 Sclerosing stromal tumors of the ovary. Cancer 31: 664–670

Damjanov I, Drobnjak P, Grizelj V, Longhino N 1975 Sclerosing stromal tumor of the ovary. Obstetrics and Gynecology 45: 675–678

Di Saia P J, Saltz A, Kagan A R, Rich W 1978 A temporary response of recurrent granulosa cell tumor to adriamycin. Obstetrics and Gynecology 52: 355–358

Evans A T, Gaffey T A, Malkasian G D, Annegers J R 1980 Clinicopathologic review of 118 granulosa and 82 theca cell tumours. Obstetrics and Gynecology 55: 231

Hart W R, Kumar N. Crissman J D 1980 Ovarian neoplasms resembling sex-cord tumors with annular tubules. Cancer 45: 2352–2363

Kurman R J, Goebelsmann U, Taylor C R 1979 Steroid localization in granulosa-theca tumors of the ovary. Cancer 43: 2377

Lomax C W, May H V, Panko W B, Thornton W N 1977 Progesterone production by an ovarian granulosa cell carcinoma. Obstetrics and Gynecology 50: 39S–40S

Lusch C J, Mercurio T M, Runyeon W K 1978 Delayed recurrence and chemotherapy of a granulosa cell tumor. Obstetrics and Gynecology 51: 505–507

Malkasian G D, Webb M J, Jorgensen E O 1974 Observations on chemotherapy of granulosa cell carcinomas and malignant ovarian teratomas. Obstetrics and Gynecology 44: 885–888

McCormack T P, Riddick D H 1976 Hormonal function of a granulosa cell tumor. Obstetrics and Gynecology 48: 16S–21S

McNatty K P, Makris A, Degrazia C, Osathanonah R, Ryan K J 1979 The production of progesterone, androgens, and estrogens by granulosa cells, thecal tissue, and stromal tissue from human ovaries in vitro. Journal of Clinical Endocrinology and Metabolism 49: 687

Meyer R 1930 Beitable zur Pathologischen Anatomie 84: 485

Norris H J, Taylor H B 1968 Prognosis of granulosa-theca tumors of the ovary. Cancer 21: 255–263

Norris H J, Taylor H B 1969 Virilization associated with cystic granulosa tumors. Obstetrics and Gynecology 34: 629–635

Novak E R, Kutchmeshgi J, Mupas R S, Woodruff J D 1971 Feminizing gonadal stromal tumors. Analysis of the granulosa-theca cell tumors of the ovarian tumor registry. Obstetrics and Gynecology 38: 701–713

Roth L M, Nicholas T R, Ehrlich C E 1979 Juvenile granulosa cell tumor. A clinicopathologic study of three cases with ultrastructural observations. Cancer 44: 2194–2205

Schwartz P E, Smith J P 1976 Treatment of ovarian stromal tumors. American Journal of Obstetrics and Gynecology 125: 402–411

Scully R E 1977 Ovarian tumors. American Journal of Pathology 87: 686

Scully R E 1970 Sex-cord tumor with annular tubules. A distinctive ovarian tumor of the Peutz-Jeghers syndrome. Cancer 25: 1107–1121

Stenwig I T, Hazenkamp J, Beecham J D 1979 Granulosa cell tumors of the ovary. A clinicopathological study of 118 cases with long-term follow-up. Gynecologic Oncology 7: 136–152

Waxman M, Vuletin J C, Urcuyo R, Belling C G 1970 Ovarian low-grade stromal sarcoma with thecomatous features. A critical reappraisal of the so-called 'malignant thecoma'. Cancer 44, 2206

16

Sertoli-Leydig and lipid cell tumours of the ovary

Introduction

Sertoli-Leydig cell tumours of the ovary are sex cord stromal tumours which contain Sertoli and Leydig cells with indifferent stroma, similar to that seen in the various phases of testicular development in the male. They represent 0.5%, and are the most commonly virilising, of all ovarian tumours. Sertoli-Leydig cell tumours are one-fifth as common as granulosa-theca cell ovarian tumours, and they occur primarily in the second and third decades, with a median age of approximately 34 years. The youngest patient reported to date, however, was two years of age. There has been a familial incidence reported, with female family members developing both Sertoli-Leydig cell tumours and thyroid adenomas (Jenson et al 1974).

In 1905, Pick first described this tumour which was later named arrhenoblastoma by Meyer, who reported 26 cases of a similar type tumour in 1931, and coined the term. He classified arrhenoblastomas into three subtypes: well-differentiated tubular adenomas, intermediate differentiated arrhenoblastomas and poorly differentiated sarcomatoid arrhenoblastomas. Telium (1958) preferred the term androblastoma to encompass all of the subtypes described by Meyer. In 1958, Morris & Scully suggested replacing the terms arrhenoblastoma or androblastoma with the term Sertoli-Leydig cell tumour to avoid the connotation that all arrhenoblastomas or androblastomas were masculinising. Although 80% of Sertoli-Leydig cell tumours are associated with virilisation, a small percentage are feminising or inert. Moreover, since there is no such cell as an arrhenoblast, and since the term arrhenoblastoma only means a tumour or 'oma', with a masculinising effect, the descriptive term Sertoli-Leydig cell tumour has replaced the term arrhenoblastoma. However, the World Health Organisation International Histologic Classification of Tumours still uses both designations — Sertoli-Leydig cell tumour and androblastoma — to describe these tumours (Serov et al 1973).

The World Health Organisation classifies Sertoli-Leydig cell tumours into four categories. The most common tumours are the well-differentiated Pick's adenoma, consisting of hollow tubules separated by Leydig cells. The intermediate differentiated tumours contain more primitive Sertoli cells arranged similarly to the sex cords of the embryonal testes. The poorly differentiated sarcomatoid tumours consist of cells resembling spindle-cell sarcoma. The fourth category is Sertoli-Leydig cell tumours with heterologous elements containing argenoffin cells, cartilage, skeletal muscle, or mucous secreting epithelium. All four categories have well-differentiated Leydig cells identical to those seen in the male testes

Differential diagnosis

The differential diagnosis of Sertoli-Leydig cell tumours includes: (1) carcinoids of the ovary, primary or metastatic, (2) testicular feminisation syndrome, (3) luteoma of pregnancy with virilisation, (4) poorly differentiated granulosa cell tumours, (5) metastatic ovarian carcinomas, (6) stromal Leydig cell tumours, (7) ovarian teratomas, (8) malignant mixed-mesodermal ovarian tumours, (9) pure Sertoli cell tumours, (10) hilus cell tumours, and (11) lipid cell tumours.

Because of the variation in histological criteria and the complexities of differential diagnosis, many of the previously reported cases of Sertoli-Leydig cell tumours or arrhenoblastomas may have been incorrectly diagnosed. This possibility is especially important when evaluating earlier reports of arrhenoblastomas in relation to treatment and survival. The variation in histological criteria and subsequent change in diagnosis on rereview was reported in a recent study by Roth and coauthors (1981). They reviewed 61 ovarian tumours that were initially diagnosed as Sertoli-Leydig cell tumours, and only 34 were found to be correctly diagnosed. The other 27 cases consisted of hamartomatous masses in the gonads in three cases of testicular feminisation, two sex cord tumours with annular tubules, five lipid tumours, two luteomas of pregnancy, four unclassified sex cord stromal tumours, one granulosa cell tumour, three carcinoid tumours, one adenocarcinoma, one poorly differentiated metastatic ovarian adenocarcinoma, one malignant mixed Mullerian tumour, one yolk sac tumour, one sarcoma and two unclassified neoplasms. Clearly, reporting all of these tumours as Sertoli-Leydig cell tumours would result in a different perception of the eventual outcome of patients with this disease.

Carcinoids may have the appearance of Sertoli-Leydig cell tumours since both have tubules or acini; however, carcinoids will have a positive argenoffin reaction. Luteomas of pregnancy can result in virilisation of the patient, but do not contain Sertoli cells. Poorly differentiated granulosa cell tumours may resemble poorly differentiated Sertoli-Leydig cell tumours, but do not contain identifiable Leydig cells. Patients with testicular feminisation syndrome may have proliferation of Sertoli and/or Leydig cells in the gonad, but there will be no normal ovarian tissue present. In addition, these patients present with primary amenorrhoea, sparse pubic and axillary hair, and no uterus. Sertoli-Leydig cell tumours can be confused with metastatic ovarian carcinoma because the acini may resemble the Sertoli cell tubule, and a hyperplastic luteinisation of the stroma, if present, may lead to mistaking these cells for Leydig cells. Moreover, the hyperplastic stroma secondary to ovarian metastasis may result in virilisation of the patient. Stromal Leydig cell tumours contain Leydig cells with crystalloids of Reinke set in an active ovarian stroma, but do not contain identifiable Sertoli cells. Since there can be heterologous elements such as mucous secreting epithelium, cartilage, skeletal muscle, and argenoffin cells present in Sertoli-Leydig cell tumours, these tumours can be confused with teratomas or malignant mixed Mullerian ovarian tumours.

Hormonal production

Virilisation in Sertoli-Leydig cell tumours is secondary to increased serum levels of testosterone. Since a small increase of serum testosterone in the female will result in significant virilisation, this increase may not be reflected in significant amounts in 24-hour urinary 17-ketosteroids. Urinary 17-ketosteroids are either normal or slightly elevated in patients with Sertoli-Leydig cell tumours. Some Sertoli-Leydig cell tumours can result in feminisation of the patient secondary to oestrogen production by the Sertoli-Leydig cell tumour itself, or by peripheral conversion from androstene-dione to oestrogen.

Survival

In 1976, Ireland & Woodruff reviewed all cases of 'masculinising ovarian tumours' entered into the Emil Novak Ovarian Tumor Registry from 1942 to 1975. The majority of cases had previously been reported as arrhenoblastomas on review by five gynaecological pathologists (Novak & Long 1965). Since the term arrhenoblastoma was felt to be inappropriate, Ireland & Woodruff reclassified these tumours into two main subclassification: gonadal stromal tumours (including arrhenoblastomas), and Sertoli-Leydig cell tumours. Of the 67 gonadal stromal tumours (including arrhenoblastoma), the tumour related mortality rate was only 7% (5). Only 4% (1) of the 23 cases reclassified as Sertoli-Leydig cell tumours had tumour related deaths. Therefore, of the 90 sex-cord stromal tumours reported by Ireland & Woodruff, the tumour-related mortality rate was 6%. This is in contrast to the report of Novak & Long who reported on 111 cases of arrhenoblastoma from the Emil Novak Ovarian Tumor Registry from 1942–1963, many of which were reclassified by Ireland & Woodruff. Of the 90 cases followed for over five years, the tumour-related mortality rate was 34% (26). This significant difference in mortality rates is a result of variation in histological criteria between the two reviews, but more importantly, Novak & Long calculated all deaths regardless of cause as death from arrhenoblastoma, rather than just tumour-related deaths.

In a report of 34 Sertoli-Leydig cell tumours by Roth et al (1981), 15 patients have been followed for more than one year, and there was one tumour-related death (6%). This is similar to the mortality rate reported by Ireland & Woodruff. Of their four patients with well-differentiated Sertoli-Leydig cell tumours followed for an average of four years, all were alive with no evidence of disease. Of the eight patients with intermediate differentiated tumours followed for an average of 7.6 years, all were alive with no evidence of disease. The only death from Sertoli-Leydig cell tumour occurred in one of the three patients with poorly differentiated disease. The latter patients were followed for an average of 4.3 years (Table 16.1).

Table 16.1 Tumour-related deaths: Sertoli-Leydig tumour (Ireland & Woodruff 1976)

Authors	Patients	Recurrences	Tumour-related deaths % (no.)
Ireland & Woodruff	67	5	7% (5)
Ireland & Woodruff	23	1	4% (1)
Roth et al	15	1	6% (1)
Total	105	7	6.6% (7)

Therefore, it would appear that the overall tumour-related mortality rate from Sertoli-Leydig cell tumours approximates 6%, or conversely, 94% of these patients will not die of the tumour. A possible exception to this statement is the mortality rate from Sertoli-Leydig cell tumours discovered in pregnant women. Galle and coauthors (1978) in a study of 200 cases, reported a case of a Sertoli-Leydig cell tumour that occurred during pregnancy at the time of initial operation, and collected 15 other cases from the literature. Of these 16 patients, seven (44%) had evidence of metastasis or recurrence, five (31%) died from Sertoli-Leydig cell tumour, and the perinatal mortality rate was 50%. However, as previously discussed, because of the variation in the histological criteria of Sertoli-Leydig cell tumours, many may not have indeed been Sertoli-Leydig cell tumours. In contrast to granulosa-theca cell tumours which may recur as late as 30 years after initial treatment, almost all examples of recurrent Sertoli-Leydig cell tumours have recurred within the first five years of initial operation.

Chemotherapy

There are only a few reports of chemotherapy for Sertoli-Leydig cell tumours because the tumour is rare, and the number of recurrences is small. Schwartz & Smith (1976) used vincristine, actinomycin-D and cyclophosphamide (VAC) in two cases of Sertoli-Leydig cell tumour and reported that both patients responded. Roth and coauthors (1981) achieved a partial response to triosulfon in a patient who did not respond initially to chlorambucil.

Treatment

The overall incidence of bilaterality of Sertoli-Leydig cell tumours is less than 5%, and in the report by Ireland & Woodruff (1976) the incidence of bilaterality was only 1%. Therefore, since most Sertoli-Leydig cell tumours occur in the second and third decades, and since the tumour-related mortality rate approximates only 6%, young patients with stage IA tumours, who desire to retain future fertility, should be treated by conservative unilateral salpingo-oophorectomy without adjuvant therapy. All other patients should be treated by hysterectomy and bilateral salpingo-oophorectomy. For patients with poorly differentiated sarcomatoid lesions, adjuvant postoperative whole abdominal irradiation or intraperitoneal ^{32}P should be considered, although there have been no data reported to support this thesis. Finally, patients with recurrent Sertoli-Leydig cell tumour who are not amenable to surgery or radiation therapy, should be treated by VAC chemotherapy.

Pure Sertoli cell ovarian tumour

The pure Sertoli ovarian tumour is of gonadal stromal origin and is composed entirely of Sertoli cells. this tumour was previously classified as a Sertoli-Leydig cell tumour even though the features of Sertoli-Leydig cell tumours, i.e., Leydig cells and primative gonadal stromal, are absent. Tavassoli & Norris (1980) reported 28 cases of pure Sertoli cell ovarian tumours from the Armed Forces Institute of Pathology. Unlike Sertoli-Leydig cell tumours, pure Sertoli cell tumours are more often associated with oestrogenic manifestations followed by virilisation. Tavassoli & Norris reported unusual hormanal manifestations in 17 of the 28 cases. Oestrogenic manifestations included isosexual precocious puberty in three prepubertal girls and menometrorrhagia in nine adult women. Virilisation occurred in four patients and was manifested by hirsutism, amenorrhoea, breast atrophy, clitoral hypertrophy and deepening of the voice. Although all 28 cases were stage IA, with no evidence of metastasis at initial operation, two patients subsequently developed recurrences, one in the pelvis and one in the peritoneal cavity. They were treated with vincristine, actinomycin-D, cyclophosphamioe and triethylenethiophosphoramide, respectively; but neither responded. Of the two neoplasms that recurred, both were larger than 10 cm, had complex tubular patterns, and had evidence of infiltration of the supporting stroma by individual neoplastic cells. Of the 28 cases, only these two neoplasms had stromal infiltration. Therefore, Tavassoli & Norris believe that stromal infiltration is the main characteristic of potentially metastatic pure Sertoli cell tumours. Treatment should consist of unilateral salpingo-oophorectomy in the younger patient desiring to retain future fertility, and hysterectomy and bilateral salpingo-oophorectomy in all other patients. Patients who do not desire future childbearing but with Sertoli tumours demonstrating stromal infiltration, should be considered for adjuvant whole abdominal irradiation or intraperitoneal ^{32}P. There is no report on the effect of chemotherapy in this disease.

Lipid cell tumours

Lipid cell tumours occur within the ovarian stroma and histologically consist of large, round, polygonal cells with vacuolated, lipid-rich cytoplasm. Microscopically, they resemble adrenal cortical, Leydig, or lutein cells. Since hilus cells, adrenal cortical cells, and luteinised ovarian stromal cells are cytologically similar, separation of these tumours into specific categories is frequently impossible. Moreover, since adrenal cortical rests have only been reported within the ovary in one instance (Symmonds & Driscoll 1973), tumours with the appearance of adrenal cortical cells or ovarian stromal tumours with the above histological appearance, but which cannot be specifically categorised, are placed within the non-specific category of lipid, or lipoid cell ovarian tumours. This tumour is almost always present in only one ovary.

Conditions often associated with virilisation that must be excluded prior to making the diagnosis of lipid cell tumour include: (1) stromal luteoma, which is a benign condition characterised by severe luteinisation of the ovarian stroma with a vacuolated lipid appearance of the luteinised cells; (2) non-hilar Leydig cells which may also display a vacuolated lipid appearance; (3) pregnancy luteoma, a condition which is characterised by the formation of nodules of lutein cells that contain little or no neutral lipid, is frequently present in both ovaries, and frequently has increased numbers of mitosis which may lead to a mistaken diagnosis of malignancy; (4) luteinised granulosa-theca cell tumours which occur primarily during pregnancy and may be confused with lipid cell tumours; (5) metastatic carcinomas to the ovary with stromal luteinisation which may cause severe luteinisation of the ovary and virilisation; however, a positive reaction for intracytoplasm mucin in metastatic carcinomas will separate these from lipid cell tumours; and (6) hilus cell tumours without cystalliods of Reinke which some authors believe cannot be specifically diagnosed as hilus cells and, therefore, are frequently included in the lipid cell tumour category.

Hormonal production

Virilisation occurred in 77% of the 30 lipid cell tumour patients reported by Taylor & Norris (1967), with hyperoestrogenism manifested in 23% (14) patients. Rice & Savard (1966) and Leymarie & Savard (1968) demonstrated that ovarian stromal cells predominantly produce androstenedione whereas hilus cells and tumours of Leydig cell origin primarily produce testosterone. Increased levels of androstenedione are reflected in increased urinary 17-ketosteroids, whereas patients with virilisation secondary to increased serum testosterone, as in Sertoli-Leydig cell tumours, hilus cell tumours and tumours of Leydig cell origin, frequently have normal or only slightly elevated urinary 17-ketosteroids. Therefore, elevated urinary 17-ketosteroids in a patient with a lipid cell ovarian tumour is helpful in separating them from Sertoli-Leydig and hilus cell tumours, and tumours of Leydig cell origin. Cushing's syndrome occurs in approximately 10% of lipid cell tumour patients, and these patients frequently have hypertension, polycythaemia and a diabetic glucose tolerance curve. However, since many of these findings are present in a significant percentage of patients without lipid cell tumours, a conclusion that these tumours are of adrenal rest origin cannot be made. Although adrenal rests do not occur within the ovary, except in possible rare cases, the recent demonstration by McGinley and coauthors (1981), of the production of a C21 steroid from a lipid cell ovarian tumour, similar to that found in the normal adrenal cortical cells, would lend credence to the theory that these adrenal cortical appearing cells are indeed adrenal in origin.

Survival

Taylor & Norris (1967) reported 30 cases of lipid cell ovarian tumours and follow-up was available on 22 patients. All tumours containing crystalloids of Reinke were proven to be benign in character, on follow-up. Of the 30 lipid tumours reported by Norris & Taylor, peritoneal metastasis was present at the time of initial operation in three patients, and in another patient, the tumour was adherent to the sigmoid colon and the greater omentum. Of the 22 patients available for follow-up, 18 had clinical stage IA disease and four had disease outside of the ovary, as described above. Three (75%) of the four patients with extra-ovarian involvement subsequently died from lipid cell tumour. Of the 18 apparent stage IA tumours, three (17%) died of the tumour. Ireland & Woodruff (1976) reported 22 cases of lipid cell ovarian tumours from the Emil Nowak Ovarian Tumor Registry which consisted of two cell populations: a larger polygonal, lipid-laden cell resembling zona fasciculata cells, and smaller cells resembling zona reticularis cells. They referred to these 22 lipid cell tumours as adrenal cortical rest tumours. Of the 18 patients on which follow-up was available, there was only one (5%) tumour-related death (Table 16.2).

Table 16.2 Survival: lipid cell tumours (Taylor & Norris 1967, Ireland & Woodruff 1976).

Authors	Patients	Stage	Tumour-related death % (no.)
Taylor & Norris	4	IIB-III	75% (3)
Taylor & Norris	18	IA	17% (3)
Ireland & Woodruff	18	IA	5% (1)

Treatment

In the 30 patients treated by Taylor & Norris (1967), the ages ranged from 19 to 78 years. In contrast, in the 22 cases reported by Ireland & Woodruff, the ages ranged from 2 to 74, but 45% of the patients were between the ages of 11 and 30, with 68% of the entire group having signs of virilisation. Of the 30 tumours reported by Taylor & Norris, all were unilateral ovarian tumours, including the four tumours with extra-ovarian involvement at initial operation. Moreover, survival was similar in their patients treated by unilateral salpingo-oophorectomy, compared to those treated with hysterectomy and bilateral salpingo-oophorectomy. Therefore, since these tumours are almost always unilateral, and frequently occur in the young patient, those desiring to retain future fertility should be treated by unilateral salpingo-oophorectomy. All other patients should be treated by hysterectomy and bilateral salpingo-oophorectomy. Patients with extra-ovarian involvement could be treated similarly to patients with Sertoli-Leydig cell tumours and extra-ovarian involvement.

Hilus cell tumours

Hilus cells are normally present in the ovarian hilus, but may be located in any part of the ovary. Like lipid cell tumours, they contain intracytoplasmic lipid inclusion. However, hilus cells are distinct from lipid cell tumours because 75% of hilus cell tumours contain crystalloids of Reinke which are characteristic of hilus and Leydig cells only, and are eosinophilic, rod-shaped structures located in the cytoplasm. When there is an increase in hilus cells, but without a definitive tumour nodule, the condition is referred to as hilus cell hyperplasia. If a tumour is present, the term hilus cell tumour is used. Previously, the diagnosis depended on the presence of crystalloids of Reinke. However, if in the mesoovarium, lipid-containing tumour cells are present, a diagnosis of hilus cell tumour can be made, especially if there is surrounding hilus cell hyperplasia.

Hilus cell tumours are rare, and to date, less than 90 cases have been reported. Of the 22 cases reported by Ireland & Woodruff (1976), the ages ranged from 11–75, with 80% of the patients being 40 years or older. They are small tumours and rarely obtain a size greater than 2 cm. To date, six cases have been associated with endometrial adenocarcinoma (Mohamed et al 1978), and six cases have been associated with polycystic ovarian disease (McBee & Stachura 1979). The cause and effect of the latter is not understood. Significant virilisation is associated with 75% of these tumours (Ireland & Woodruff 1976), and all virilised patients have significant hirsutism. A smaller percentage have signs of hyperoestrogenism as manifested by postmenopausal bleeding, menorrhagia, endometrial hyperplasia, or even, endometrial adenocarcinoma. The cases associated with virilism have demonstrated a significant increase of serum testosterone and normal to slightly elevated urinary 17-ketosteroids. Occasionally, virilised patients will have normal appearing ovaries, but selective catheterisation of the ovarian veins will demonstrate increased levels of testosterone and resection of the ovary will show a small hilus cell tumour.

There is some debate as to whether a malignant hilus cell tumour has ever been reported (Echt & Hadd 1968). Almost all are unilateral and most authors consider them to be a benign tumour. However, possibly many of the lipid cell tumours, which do not have Reinke crystalloids, and which have acted in the malignant fashion, may indeed have been malignant hilus cell tumours.

Survival and treatment

There were no tumour-related deaths of the 22 cases reported by Ireland & Woodruff (1976) from the Emil Novak Ovarian Tumor Registry.

Since most authors agree that there has been no convincing report of a clinically malignant hilus cell tumour, all young patients should be treated by unilateral salpingo-oophorectomy. Older patients should be treated by hysterectomy and bilateral salpingo-oophorectomy.

Stromal Leydig cell tumour

Stromal Leydig cell tumours are rare and occur in the ovarian stroma. They consist of Leydig cells in a nodular formation and contain characteristic Reinke crystalloids. Sex-cord stromal elements such as Sertoli or granulosa cells are not present. In addition to the characteristic Leydig cells, there are spindle-shaped stromal cells present, which are distinct from the stromal luteomas. These virilising stromal Leydig cell tumours have been reported only on very rare occasions; all have occurred in perimenopausal women and all were benign. They resemble luteinised theca cell tumours except the Leydig cells are present. The tumour may produce virilisation, but is rarely associated with increased oestrogen production.

REFERENCES

Echt C R, Hadd H E 1968 Androgen excretion patterns in a patient with a metastatic hilus cell tumour of the ovary. American Journal of Obstetrics and Gynecology 100: 1055

Galle P C, McCool J A, Elsner C W 1978 Arrhenoblastoma during pregnancy. Obstetrics and Gynecology 51: 3, 359

Imperato-McGinley J, Peterson R E, Dawood M Y et al 1981 Steroid hormone secretion from a virilising lipoid cell tumour of the ovary. Obstetrics and Gynecology 57: 525

Sertoli Leydig and lipid cell tumours of the ovary

Ireland K, Woodruff J D 1976 Review: masculinising ovarian tumours. Obstetrics and Gynecology Survey 31: 2, 83

Jenson R D, Norris H J, Fraumeni J F, Jr. 1974 Familial arrhenoblastoma and thyroid adenoma. Cancer 33: 218

Leymarie P, Savard K 1968 Steroid hormone formation in the human ovary. VI. Evidence for two pathways of synthesis of androgens in the stromal compartment. Journal of Clinical Endocrinology 28: 1547

McBee A, Stachura I 1979 Case report: ovarian hilar cell tumour with co-existent polycystic ovary syndrome and myometrial hypertrophy. Gynecologic Oncology 8: 370

Meyer R 1931 Pathology of some special ovarian tumours and their relation to sex characteristics. American Journal of Obstetrics and Gynecology 22: 697

Mohamed N C, Cardenas A, Villasanta U, et al 1978 Hilus cell tumour of the ovary and endometrial carcinoma. Obstetrics and Gynecology 52: 486

Morris J M, Scully R E 1958 Endocrine pathology of the ovary. Mosby, St Louis p 89

Novak E R, Long J H 1965 Arrhenoblastoma of the ovary. American Journal of Obstetrics and Gynecology 92: 8, 1082

Pick L 1905 Ueber abenome der mannlichen und weiblichen keimdruse bei hermaphoroditismus verus and spurius. Klinische Wochenschrift 42: 502

Rice B F, Savard K 1966 Steroid hormone formation in the human ovary: IV. Ovarian stromal compartment, formation of radioactive steroids from acetate ^{14}Cl-C and action of gonadotropins. Journal of Clinical Endocrinology 26: 593

Roth L M, Anderson M C, Govan A D T et al 1981 Sertoli-Leydig cell tumours: a clinicopathologic study of 34 cases. Cancer 48: 187–197

Schwartz P E, Smith J P 1976 Treatment of ovarian stromal tumours. American Journal of Obstetrics and Gynecology 125: 402

Serov S F, Scully R E, Sobin R H 1973 Histological typing of ovarian tumours. International Histologic Classification of Tumours, 9, Geneva: World Health Organization

Symmonds D A, Driscoll S G 1973 An adrenal cortical rest within a fetal ovary. Report of a case. American Journal of Clinical Pathology 60: 562

Tavassoli F A, Norris H J 1980 Sertoli tumours of the ovary. A clinicopathologic study of 28 cases with ultrastructural observations. Cancer 46: 2281

Taylor H B, Norris H J 1967 Lipid cell tumours of the ovary. Cancer 29: 1953

Teilum G 1958 Classification of testicular and ovarian androblastoma and Sertoli cell tumours. A survey of comparative studies with consideration of histogenesis, endocrinology, and embryological theories. Cancer 11: 769

17

Ovarian sarcomas

Introduction

Ovarian sarcomas are rare, accounting for less than 1% of all ovarian malignancies. Of 2400 cases of ovarian malignancies reported in the Emil Novak Ovarian Tumor Registry, only 43 were primarily ovarian sarcomas (Azoury & Woodruff 1971). Ovarian sarcomas occur primarily in postmenopausal women of low parity. They grow rapidly and most patients present with abdominal masses at the initial examination. Most ovarian sarcoma patients die within two years of diagnosis. The high mortality rate results from the fact that there is metastasis beyond the pelvis in over 80% of the patients at the initial examination, and that to date, there is no effective chemotherapy to control this spread.

Since embryologists exclude the ovary as being of Mullerian derivative, the histogenesis of ovarian sarcomas remains debatable. They are not teratomatous in origin because there are no germ cells present from which teratomas are normally derived. It is important, however, to differentiate ovarian sarcomas from ovarian teratomas, since ovarian teratomas occur in a younger age group, and since high cure rates have been obtained by conservative surgery and adjuvant chemotherapy. Many believe that ovarian sarcomas arise from endometriosis. However, endometriosis is not normally present in the age group that develops ovarian sarcomas, and the association of endometriosis and this malignancy has been demonstrated in less than one in ten cases. Others have postulated the coelomic epithelium metaplastic theory, i.e., ovarian sarcomas have a mesodermal origin.

Although the histogenesis is debatable and there is no current classification of ovarian sarcomas, for clinical purposes they can be grouped into four main types: (1) adenosarcomas which are low-grade sarcomas characterised by an intermixture of non-malignant glandular elements and stromal sarcoma components; (2) carcinosarcomas which consist of carcinomatous and non-specific homologous mesenchymal sarcoma elements; (3) mixed mesodermal tumours or mixed mesodermal sarcomas which contain heterologous stromal components of cartilage, bone, adipose tissue or striated muscle; and (4) fibrosarcomas.

Adenosarcomas

Adenosarcomas have a low malignancy potential and a tendency for local recurrence. In 1974, Clement & Scully described the first cases of uterine adenosarcomas which consisted of an intimate admixture of sarcomatous stromal elements resembling endometrial stromal sarcoma, and benign, but often atypical, epithelial elements. Later, these authors (Clement & Scully 1977) described the first two cases of ovarian adenosarcomas which were low-grade sarcomas associated with local pelvic recurrences and long-term survival. Kao & Norris (1978) reported 11 cases of adenosarcoma of the ovary and adnexal region. Of the five lowest grade tumours, all were confined to the ovary, and did not recur after surgical excision, whereas two of the three intermediate grade neoplasms extended beyond the ovary, but were arrested by combination chemotherapy.

Carcinosarcomas

Recently, Ober (1979) collected 77 cases of ovarian carcinosarcoma from a review of the literature. The median age was 60 and only 20% occurred in patients less than 50 years of age. Most patients were nulliparous and presented with an abdominal mass, after only a short history of abnormal symptoms. Only three (4%) of the 77 cases survived five years, and two-thirds died in less than 18 months. Fenn & Abell (1971) reported 23 cases of ovarian carcinosarcoma. Twenty-two of these patients died and one survived (144 months), at the time of their report. Of the 22 patients that died, only one had survived longer than two years.

Mixed mesodermal tumour or mixed mesodermal sarcoma

Hernadez and coauthors (1977) reviewed 90 cases of mixed mesodermal tumour reported in the literature and added three new cases. These tumours occurred primarily in the sixth and seventh decades, with a median age of 58. Fifty-two per cent (47) of the women died less than six months after the initial surgery, and 77% (69) died in less than 12 months. Only 29% (7) of the 24 stage I patients survived for more than two years. Of the 50 stage III women, 74% (37) died less than six months after diagnosis.

Fibrosarcomas

Most fibromatous ovarian tumours are benign and have only rare mitosis. Occasionally, there are fibromatous tissues with increased mitosis and these are designated as fibrosarcomas. They are characterised by hypercellularity, high mitotic rate and marked nuclear pleomorphism. Prat & Scully (1981) analysed 17 cases of fibromatous ovarian tumours in an attempt to separate cellular fibromas from fibrosarcomas. The first group, consisting of 11 patients with cellular fibromas, were alive and well from 33 months to 13 years. The only cellular fibroma patient who died of recurrent tumour had incomplete resection of a primary tumour that was attached to the omentum and pelvic wall at the time of initial surgery. The other case of cellular fibroma that recurred, did so seven years after initial surgery but there had been a rupture of the tumour at the initial operation. The second group consisted of six fibrosarcomas with four or more mitosis per 10 high-power fields, and grade 2 to 3 nuclear pleomorphism. The fibrosarcomas all pursued an aggressive course with four of the six patients dead two months to four years after the initial operation.

Treatment

Stage I ovarian sarcomas

As noted, the prognosis for ovarian sarcomas, except for adenosarcomas, remains very poor. Other than surgical resection, very little has been achieved by adjuvant radiation or chemotherapy. However, Smith and coauthors (1975) reported that radiation followed by vincristine, actinomycin-D and cyclophosphamide

(VAC) chemotherapy was effective in pelvic sarcomas in general, four of which were primary ovarian sarcomas. Patients received 2600–2800 rads to the entire abdomen by the moving strip technique, followed by an additional 2000 rads to the whole pelvis and the VAC chemotherapy. This therapy may result in improved survival for patients with clinically localised ovarian sarcomas who were initially treated by hysterectomy and bilateral salpingo-oophorectomy.

Since the reported cases of adenosarcomas that have recurred are rare, and have only occurred locally in the pelvis, the adjuvant use of whole pelvis irradiation (5000 rads in 5–5.5 weeks) should result in a decreased incidence of local recurrence and improved survival.

Stage II, III & IV ovarian sarcomas

Patients with large residual disease require systemic chemotherapy. Of the 1275 ovarian cancer cases treated from 1968–1979, at Roswell Park Memorial Institute, 35 (2.6%) were primary ovarian sarcomas (Lele et al 1980). All 35 women were treated with chemotherapy (Table 17.1). Nine women received first, second and third-line VAC chemotherapy, and two patients responded, one completely and one partially (Table 17.2). The most effective chemotherapy for soft tissue and bone sarcomas has been cyclophosphamide, vincristine, adriamycin and imidazole carboxamide (CYVADIC). Gottlieb and coauthors (1975) reported a 55% response rate to CYVADIC in 136 women with soft tissue and bone sarcomas, making this chemotherapy combination the most effective for sarcomas in general. We have treated 26 pelvic sarcoma patients with CYVADIC and 23% have responded (Piver et al 1981). However, none of the four ovarian sarcoma patients treated with CYVADIC responded (Lele et al 1980). Of the other five combinations tried (high-dose methotrexate plus cyclophosphamide; actinomycin-D, 5-fluorouracil and cyclosphosphamide (ACFUCY); actinomycin-D, 5-fluorouracil and melphalan; methotrexate, adriamycin and cyclophosphamide (MAC); cis-platinum and imidazole carboxamide), three patients responded, including a complete response to ACFUCY, a partial response to MAC, and a partial response to third-line cis-platinum and imidazole carboxamide. None of the 13 patients who received single-agent chemotherapy responded.

Table 17.1 Chemotherapy regimens

Abbreviation	Drugs	Dose	Length of Cycle
1. ADR	Adriamycin	45 mg/m²/day/i.v. × 2	2 day course repeated every 4 weeks
2.	Melphalan	0.2 mg/kg/day p.o. × 5	5 day course repeated every 4 weeks
3.	Prednimustin	20 mg/day/p.o.	daily continuously
4. MCCNU	Methyl MCCNU	150 g/m²/once	repeated every 6 weeks
5.	Thiotepa	30–45 mg/i.v. once a week	weekly
6.	Cyclophosphamide	100 mg/day	daily continuously
7. HDMTX + CTX	Methotrexate	750 mg/m²/i.v. –4 hrs/day one only	
	Leukovorin	10 mg/m²/every 6 hrs/i.m. × 12	5 day course repeated every 4 weeks
8. MAC	Cyclophosphamide	7 mg/kg/day × 5	
	Methotrexate	750 mg/m²/i.v.–4 hrs, day 1 only	
	Leukovorin	10 mg/²q 6 h × 12	
	Cyclophosphamide	200 mg/m²/i.v. daily × 5	
9. ACFUCY	Adriamycin	40 g/m²/day 4	
	Actinomycin-D	0.5 mg/day/i.v. × 5	
	5FU	8 mg/kg/day/i.v. × 5	5 day course repeated every 4 weeks
	Cyclophosphamide	7 mg/kg/day/i.v. × 5	5 day course repeated every 4 weeks
10. ACFUME	Actinomycin-D	0.5 mg/day/i.v. × 5	
	5FU	8 mg/kg/day i.v. × 5	5 day course repeated every 4 weeks
	Melphalan	0.1 mg/kg/day/p.o. × 5	
11. VAC	Vincristine	1.5 mg/m²/week = 2 mg or less	every week × 12
	Actinomycin-D	0.5 mg/day/i.v. × 5	
	Cyclophosphamide	7 mg/kg/day/i.v. × 5	5 day course repeated every 4 weeks
12. ADR + DTIC	Adriamycin	60 mg/m²/i.v./day 1 only	
	DTIC	100 mg/m²/i.v./daily × 5	5 day course repeated every 4 weeks
13. PLAT + DTIC	Platinum	1 mg/kg/i.v. over 6 hrs.	5 day course repeated every 4 weeks
	DTIC	200 g/m²/daily × 5	
14. CY-VA-DIC	Cyclophosphamide	400 mg/m² on day 2 i.v.	
	Vincristine	1 mg/m² on day 1 and 5 i.v.	
	Adriamycin	40 mg/m² on day 2 i.v.	5 day course repeated every 4 weeks
	DTIC	200 mg/m²/daily × 5 i.v.	

Table 17.2 Response of ovarian sarcomas to chemotherapy regimens (Lele et al 1980)

Chemotherapy	Response	First Line				Second Line				Third Line				Total			
		C	P	S	PR	C	P	S	PR	C	P	S	PR	C	P	S	PR
VAC	2/9	1	0	2	3	0	1	0	1	0	0	0	1	1	1	2	5
ADR + DTIC	0/9	0	0	0	1	0	0	0	8	0	0	0	0	0	0	0	9
HDMTX + CTX	0/6	0	0	3	0	0	0	1	1	0	0	0	1	0	0	4	2
MAC	1/1	0	1	0	0	0	0	0	0	0	0	0	0	0	1	0	0
PLAT + DTIC	1/1	0	0	0	0	0	0	0	0	0	1	0	0	0	1	0	0
ACFUCY	1/2	1	0	0	1	0	0	0	0	0	0	0	0	1	0	0	1
ACFUME	0/1	0	0	0	1	0	0	0	0	0	0	0	0	0	0	0	1
ADR	0/2	0	0	1	0	0	0	0	1	0	0	0	0	0	0	1	1
Melphalan	0/6	0	0	2	3	0	0	0	0	0	0	0	1	0	0	2	4
Cyclophosphamide	0/1	0	0	0	1	0	0	0	0	0	0	0	0	0	0	0	1
Thiotepa	0/1	0	0	0	1	0	0	0	0	0	0	0	0	0	0	0	1
Prednimustin	0/2	0	0	0	2	0	0	0	0	0	0	0	0	0	0	0	2
CCNU	0/1	0	0	0	0	0	0	0	0	0	0	0	1	0	0	0	1
TOTAL	5/42	2	1	8	13	0	1	1	11	0	1	0	4	2	3	9	28

C = complete response   P = partial response   S = stationary disease   PR = progression

To date, VAC chemotherapy seems to be the most effective combination of a largely ineffective group of combinations. A further evaluation of CYVADIC chemotherapy should be carried out because of its high activity in other sarcomas.

This book, chapter, page, paragraph and sentence, ends with the ovarian malignancy (sarcoma) that exhibits the worst prognosis and in which the least progress has been achieved. However, because of the significant progress in the past decade made in the treatment of the other 28 malignancies discussed in this book, it is hopeful, and even predicted, that improved therapy will be discovered in the not too distant future for women with this highly malignant tumour — ovarian sarcoma.

REFERENCES

Azoury R S, Woodruff J D 1971 Primary ovarian sarcomas. Report of 43 cases from the Emil Novak Ovarian Tumor Registry. Obstetrics and Gynecology 37: 918–941

Clement P B, Scully R E 1977 Extrauterine mesodermal (Mullerian) adenosarcoma. A clinicopathologic analysis of five cases. American Society of Clinical Pathology 59: 276–283

Clement P B, Scully R E 1974 Mullerian adenosarcoma of the uterus. A clinicopathologic analysis of 10 cases of a distinctive type of Mullerian mixed tumor. Cancer 34: 1138

Fenn M E, Abell M R 1971 Carcinosarcoma of the ovary. American Journal of Obstetrics and Gynecology 110: 1066–1074

Gottlieb J A, Baker L H, O'Bryan R M et al 1975 Adriamycin (NSC–123127) used alone and in combination for soft tissue and bone sarcomas. Cancer Chemotherapy Reports 6: 271–282

Hernandez W, Di Saia P J, Marrow C P, Townsend D E 1977 Mixed mesodermal sarcoma of the ovary. Obstetrics and Gynecology 49: 59s–63s

Kao G F, Norris H J 1978 Benign and low-grade variants of mixed mesodermal tumor (adenosarcoma) of the ovary and adnexal region. Cancer 42: 1314–1324

Lele S B, Piver M S, Barlow J J 1980 Chemotherapy in management of mixed mesodermal tumors of the ovary. Gynecologic Oncology 10: 298–302

Ober W B 1979 Carcinosarcoma of the ovary. Case report, review of literature, and comment on the subcoelomic mesenchyme. American Journal of Diagnostic Gynecology and Obstetrics 1: 73–81

Piver S, DeEulis T, Lele S B, Barlow J J 1981 Cyclophosphamide, vincristine, adriamycin, and imidazole carboxamide (CYVADIC) in sarcoma of the female genital tract. Gynecologic Oncology (In Press)

Pratt J, Scully R E 1981 Cellular fibromas ano fibrosarcomas of the ovary: a comparative clinicopathologic analysis of seventeen cases. Cancer 47: 2663–2670

Smith J P, Rutledge F 1975 Advances in chemotherapy for gynecologic cancer. Cancer 36: 669–674

Index

ACFUCY combination chemotherapy, 104, 110, 113, 139, 176, 180, 197, 198, 199
ACFUME combination chemotherapy, 198, 199
Actinomycin-D, 104, 110, 112, 130, 139, 140, 150–151, 153, 154, 157, 161, 180, 186, 187, 197, 198, 199, 200
Adenosarcomas, 195
ADR combination chemotherapy, 198, 199
ADR + DTIC combination chemotherapy, 198, 199
Adrenal cortical rest tumours, 43, 188
Adriamycin, 100, 103, 105, 106, 110–114, 175–176, 180, 197, 198
Age and differential diagnosis, 62
Alkeran see Melpheran
Alkylating agents, 99–108, 116–117
Alpha-1-antitrypsin, 46
Alpha-fetoprotein (AFP), 13–14, 46, 48, 136, 142, 143
Alpha-L-fucosidase, 16
Amethopterane see Methotrexate
Anaplastic dysgerminoma, 150
Androblastoma see Sertoli-Leydig cell tumours
Androgen production, 59–60, 170, 178
Antigens, 10–17
Argenoffin, 183, 184
Argentaffin, 52, 53, 59, 160
Argyrophil, 52, 53, 59, 160
Arrhenoblastoma see Sertoli-Leydig cell tumours
Asbestos, 1–2
Ascites, 6, 37, 123, 164

Beta-oncofetoprotein (BOFA), 14
Bilaterality, 63–64, 69, 147
Bjorklund isoenzyme, 12
Bleomycin, 141–142, 143, 151, 157,

Borderline malignancy, 21, 32–33, 68–73, 123–124
Bradykinin, 160
Breast carcinoma, 3, 57, 58
Brenner tumours, 32–33, 122–126
Burkitt lymphoma, 59

Call-Exner bodies, 35, 170
Carcinoembryonic antigen (CEA), 13
Carcinoid syndrome, 159–160, 161
Carcinoids, primary, 52–53, 159–162
   metastatic, 58–59, 159–162
Carcinomas, metastatic, 57–59, 63–64
Carcinoplacental antigens, 11–12
Carcinosarcomas, 195
Catecholamines, 160
CHAD (CHAP) combination chemotherapy, 105–106, 111, 112–113, 114
Chemotherapy, 104–108
   and second look laparotomy, 117–120
   choriocarcinomas, 154–155, 157
   dysgerminomas, 150
   granulosa-theca cell tumours, 175–176
   immature teratomas, 130–133
   sarcomas, 196–200
   Sertoli-Leydig cell tumours, 186
   stage I and II carcinomas, 91–97
   stage III and IV adenocarcinomas, 99–114
Chlorambucil, 99, 100, 139, 150
Choriocarcinoma, 48, 60, 136, 153–157
Chromic phosphate, 84–91, 97, 187, 188
Cis-dichlorodiamine (Cis-platinum), 100, 103–106, 110–114, 141–142, 143, 197, 198
Clear cell tumours, 31–32
CMF combination chemotherapy, 104
Coffee bean nuclei, 169

Common epithelial tumours, 19–34
Computerised axial tomography (CAT), 8
Contraception, 3
Cortisol, 43
Cushing's syndrome, 43, 189
Cyclophosphamide, 99, 100, 104–106, 110–114, 130, 139, 151, 157, 161, 176, 180, 186, 187, 196–199
Cystadenocarcinoma, 13
Cystic granulosa-cell tumours, 173, 179
Cysts, dermoid, 49–51
   tumour-like, 61–62
Cytological washings, malignant, 6, 75, 78, 79, 80, 81, 119–120
Cytoxin *see* Cyclophosphamide
CYVADIC combination chemotherapy, 197, 198, 200

Debulking surgery, 106–108
Dermoid cysts, 49–51
Diagnosis, 159–162, 168–170, 183–184
   early, 5–17
   preoperative and postoperative, 62–65
Diaphragmatic metastasis, 75, 76, 79, 80, 81, 84, 93, 121
Diethylstilboestrol, 32
Doxorubicin *see* Adriamycin
Dysgerminoma, 45–46, 60, 145–152

Embryonal carcinoma, 47–48, 60, 135–143
Endodermal sinus tumours, 14, 46–47, 135–143
Endometrial adenocarcinoma, 177, 191
Endometrial carcinoma, 3, 58
Endometrial hyperplasia, 123, 172, 177, 178
Endometrioid tumours, 28–30
Endometriosis, 32, 194
Endometriotic cysts, 62
Endoxan *see* Cyclophosphamide
Epithelial tumours, common, 19–34
Extraembryonal teratoma *see* Embryonal carcinoma; Endodermal sinus tumour

Fallopian tube carcinomas, 58
Familial incidence, 4–5, 182
Fetal antigens, 13–14
Fetal ferritin, 14
Fibrin degradation products (FDP), 16
Fibroma tumours, 36–38, 167

Fibrosarcomas, 196
Fibrothecomas, 38, 167
FIGO staging system, 6
5-Fluorouracil (5FU), 100, 103, 104, 105, 110, 112, 151, 176, 180, 197, 198

Galactosyltransferase, 16
Germ-cell tumours, 45–53
   mixed, 54–56, 153, 155–157
Germinomas, 54–56
Gestational ovarian choriocarcinoma, 155
Gold, radioactive (^{198}Au), 71, 84, 85, 89–90, 91
Gonadal neoplasia, 54–56
Gonadoblastomas, 55–56
Granulosa cell tumours, 34–36, 167–180
Gynandroblastoma, 40–41, 167, 179

HAD combination chemotherapy, 105, 111, 112–113, 114
HC combination chemotherapy, 104
HD combination chemotherapy, 112
HDMTX + CTX combination chemotherapy, 198, 199
HEXACAF combination chemotherapy, 104, 105, 106–107
Hexamethylmelamine (HXM), 100, 103, 104, 105, 110–114
Hilus cell tumours, 44, 191–192
Histamine, 160
Hobnail cells, 31–32
Hormonal aetiology, 3
Hormonal production, 168, 171–173, 184–185, 187, 189, 191
Human chorionic gonadotrophin (HCG), 12, 48, 59–60, 136, 146, 153, 154, 155
Human placental lactogen (HPL), 12
Hydrothorax, 37, 123
Hypercalcaemia, 33
Hyperreactio luteinalis, 61
Hyperthyroidism, 52, 163–164

Ileal metastasis, 58–59
Imidazole carboxamide, 197
Immature ovarian teratomas, 49, 128–133
Immunodiagnosis, 10–17
Immunoperoxidase, 136
Insular carcinoids, 52, 159, 160–162
Intestine, 121
Iodine, radioactive (^{131}I), 164, 165

Irradiation
  intraperitoneal, 84–91, 97, 164, 165, 187
  pelvic, 71, 83, 91–97, 125, 149, 197
  whole abdominal, 91–97, 117, 147–152, 196–197
Isoenzymes, 11–12

Juvenile granulosa-theca cell tumours, 173, 179

Krukenberg tumours, 9, 57–58, 63

Laparoscopy, diagnostic, 8–9
  second-look, 119–121
Laparotomy, staging, 74–81
  second-look, 116–121
Laterality, 63–64, 69, 147
Leukaemia, acute nonlymphocytic, 116–117
Leukeran see Chlorambucil
Leukovorin, 198
Leydig cell hyperplasia, 123
Leydig cell tumours, 44–45, 167
Lipid cell tumours, 42–45, 188–191
Liver, 6, 164
Luteinised thecoma, 37
Lymphomas, ovarian, 59

MAC combination chemotherapy
  with actinomycin-D, 150–151, 154–155, 157
  with adriamycin, 197, 198, 199
MCCNU combination chemotherapy, 198, 199
MECY combination chemotherapy, 105
Meigs syndrome, 37, 123, 124, 126
Melphalan, 94, 95, 96, 97, 99–104, 105–106, 110, 117, 175–176, 180, 198, 199
Menstrual disturbances, 48
Mesoblastoma see Embryonal carcinoma; Endodermal sinus tumour
Mesodermal sarcomas, 196
Mesonephroid tumours see Clear cell tumours
Metastasis, 6, 74–81
Metastatic carcinoids, 58–59, 159–162
Metastatic ovarian tumours, 57–59, 63–64
Methotrexate, 100, 103, 104, 105, 106, 112, 139, 150, 151, 153, 154, 155, 157, 197, 198

Methyl MCCNU, 198
Mixed epithelial tumours, 34
Monodermal (monophyletic) teratomas, 49, 51–53, 159–165
Mucinous tumours, 26–28
Mumps, 3

Nagao isoenzyme, 12
Neuroectodermal malignant tumours, 53
Nuclear grooves, 169, 170

Oedema, massive, 62
Oestrogen production, 3, 4, 40, 42, 59–60, 171–172, 177, 178, 187
Omental metastasis, 74, 75, 77–78, 79, 80, 81, 84, 121
Ovarian cancer antigen (OCA), 15
Ovarian cystadenocarcinoma associated antigen (OCAA), 15–16

PAC combination chemotherapy, 105
Para-aortal nodal metastasis, 76–77, 79, 80, 81, 84, 121
Pelvic node metastasis, 79, 80–81, 84, 121
Peritoneal washings, malignant, 6, 75, 78–79, 80, 81, 119–120
Peutz-Jeghers syndrome, 42, 178
L-phenylalanine see Melphalan
Phosphorus, radioactive (^{32}P), 84–91, 97, 187, 188
Pick's adenoma, 183
Placental alkaline phosphatases, 11–12
Placental hormones, 12, 48, 59–60, 136, 146, 153, 154, 155
PLAT + DTIC combination chemotherapy, 198, 199
Platinum see Cis-dichlorodiamine
Polycystic ovarian disease, 146, 191
Polyembryoma, 48, 60
Prednimustin, 198, 199
Pregnancy, 2–3, 60, 61, 146
  luteomas, 44, 61
  specific glycoprotein (SP$_1$), 12
  test positive, 136
Preoperative tests, 9–10
Primary carcinoids, 52–53, 159–162
Progesterone production, 59–60, 171–172
Proliferative Brenner tumours, 32–33, 123–124

Index

Pseudomyxoma peritonei, 28
Pyridoxine, 112, 113

Radiotherapy *see* Irradiation
Regan isoenzyme, 11
Reinke, crystalloids of, 44, 189, 191, 192
Retinal anlage tumours, 53
Rotikansky protuberance, 50

Sarcomas, 194–200
Schiller-Duval bodies, 46, 47, 136
Sclerosing stromal tumours, 38, 167, 177–178, 179
Sebaceous gland neoplasms, 53
Second-look laparoscopy, 119–121
laparotomy, 116–121
Seminomas, 54–55
Serotonin, 160
Serous tumours, 21–26
Sertoli cell adenomas, 167
Sertoli cell tumours, 167, 187–188
Sertoli-Leydig cell tumours, 38–40, 167, 182–187
Serum markers, 10–17
Sex cord-stromal tumours, 34–42, 54–56, 167–180
unclassified, 41–42, 167, 177–178
Sex cord tumour with annular tubules (SCTAT), 178
Sexual abnormality, 54–56
see also Virilisation
Staging laparotomy, 74–81
Staging system (FIGO), 6
Stein-Leventhal syndrome, 62
Steroid cell tumours, 44–45
Steroid production, 168, 171–173, 184–185, 187, 189, 191
Stromal hyperplasia, 61
Stromal hyperthecosis, 61–62
Stromal leutinisation, 123
Stromal Leydig cell tumours, 192
Stromal luteoma, 44
Struma ovarii, 51–52, 164–165
Strumal carcinoids, 53, 159, 163–164
Symptomatology, 6–7

Talc, 1–2
Teilum tumour *see* Endodermal sinus tumour

Teratomas, 48–53
immature, 49, 128–133
mature, 49–51
monodermal (monophyletic), 49, 51–53, 159–165
Testicular feminisation, 54, 147
Thecafibromas, 38, 167
Thecoma tumours, 36–38, 167, 176–177, 179
Thiotepa, 99, 100, 101, 110, 176, 187, 198, 199
Thyroid acini, 163–164
Thyroid hyperfunction, 52, 53, 164, 165
Trabecular carcinoids, 52, 159, 162–163
Triethylenethiophosphoramide (Thiotepa), 99, 100, 101, 110, 176, 187, 198, 199
Triosulphon, 186
Trophoblastic elements, 59–60
Tubo-ovarian carcinoma, 58
Tumour-associated antigens, 14–16
Tumour-like conditions, 60–62
Tumour markers, 10–17
Turner's syndrome, 146

Ultrasonography, 8
Undifferentiated carcinoma, 33

VAC combination chemotherapy, 130, 132, 133, 139, 151, 161, 186, 187, 198, 199
VBP combination chemotherapy, 141–142, 143, 151, 157
Vinblastine, 141–142, 143, 151, 157
Vincristine, 130, 139, 151, 157, 161, 186, 187, 197, 198
Virilisation, 55, 60, 62, 68, 146, 163, 173, 184–185, 188, 189, 191, 192

WHO classification of ovarian tumours, 22–23

Yolk sac tumour (endodermal sinus tumour), 14, 46–47, 135–143